THE PROBLEM
OF STUTTERING:
Theory and Therapy

Edited by

R.W. Rieber

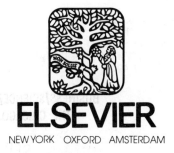

ELSEVIER

NEW YORK   OXFORD   AMSTERDAM

Elsevier North-Holland, Inc.
52 Vanderbilt Avenue, New York, New York 10017

Elsevier Scientific Publishing Company
335 Jan Van Galenstraat, P.O. Box 211
Amsterdam, The Netherlands

Library of Congress Cataloging in Publication Data

Main entry under title:

The Problem of stuttering: theory and therapy.

    "Most of these papers were originally presented
at the Second Annual Emil Froeschels Conference on
Communication Disorders held at Pace University in
New York City, January 1975."
    Includes index.
    CONTENTS: Current theory and therapy for
stuttering. Rieber, R.W. and Wollock, J. The
historical routes of the theory and therapy of
stuttering. Murphy, A.T. Authenticity and
creativity in stuttering theory and therapy.
Wingate, M.E. [etc.]
    1. Stuttering–Congresses. I. Rieber,
Robert W. II. Froeschels, Emil, 1884–
III. Emil Froeschels Conference on Communication
Disorders, 2d, Pace University, 1975. [DNLM:
1. Stuttering–Congresses. 2. Stuttering–History–Congresses. W3 EM53 1975p / WM475 E534 1975p]
RC 424.P94   616.8'554   77-4910
ISBN 0-444-00222-7

Manufactured in the United States of America

The Problem of Stuttering

To the memory of my teacher and friend,
Emil Froeschels

FOREWORD

Stuttering is the great white whale of speech disorders. The longest sought in the most remote reaches by numerous and dedicated if not obsessed pursuers, it continues to thwart those who have the audacity to contend with it. Stuttering keeps its secret. In its own way, however, it instructs, informs, and ultimately educates, refines and enlightens the frustrated souls who study it. This is nowhere as apparent as in the pages of this book. Here is the record of an exchange of views by a number of professionals who have given a large part of their working time, along with a good measure of wisdom, humanity, and wit, to the problem of stuttering. Most of us who read this document will probably be students or speech pathologists with prior knowledge of the subject. It is a fascinating exercise to imagine ourselves studying its contents through the eyes of someone comparatively uninformed about stuttering. What impressions would such a person gain about stuttering, about those who struggle with it, and about the kind of activity in which they engage?

To begin with, there are the monumental contradictions that preclude any simple outlook on the problem and make it so intractable. To speak fluently is such an easy accomplishment for most stutterers that they almost always seem just a short step away from becoming normal speakers. Yet once they have begun to speak normally they seem to be almost continually under the threat of imminent relapse. As a result, stuttering can give the bewildering impression of being at once remarkably easy and very difficult to treat. In our groping toward an effective approach to therapy, we seem to value nothing as much as a new method, unless it is one that is very old. That is, we properly distrust every measure that seems to us to be "traditional" until it becomes all but extinct, and then we revive the suffering old bag of bones with an enthusiastic whack and march it off to replace the point of view that has most lately become traditional. In this way the new often becomes old and the old new with a whimsy that can be startling to all but those who have just arrived on the scene.

This is true of our theories as well. Few of them are really new, and some of the most recent of them bear a striking resemblance to notions that were old before the end of the nineteenth century. But of all the inconsistencies of stuttering perhaps the most troublesome is the one that was referred to many decades ago by a discouraged writer—we have forgotten his name—who said, "The stutterer himself will eventually disprove every generalization we try to assert about the disorder." This is unfortunately still the case.

There is another valid impression about our prolonged quest for the cause and cure of stuttering that is amply conveyed by this book. As we read the literature on stuttering it sometimes seems as though there is hardly a major area of modern thought or study to which researchers on stuttering have not turned at some time. Our writings on the subject abound in the technical terminology of medicine, physiology, genetics, anthropology, sociology, linguistics, and almost every branch and twig of psychology. For the sake of new outlooks on stuttering we have scaled the heights of psychoanalysis, general semantics, learning theory, cybernetics, and transformational grammar. We have sat at the feet of Freud, Hull, Skinner, and Chomsky. The study of stuttering has become a university. Hardly an important intellectual impulse of value in the study of man has failed to find a place in it. Perhaps this is what one observer meant when he wrote a long time ago that the person who finds a cure for stuttering will probably find a remedy for all the ills of humankind.

OLIVER BLOODSTEIN
Brooklyn College, CUNY

Contents

continued on following page

EDITOR'S INTRODUCTION

In this volume, our readers will find some of the more representative contemporary views on both theory and therapy of stuttering. Most of these papers were originally presented at the Second Annual Emil Froeschels Conference on Communication Disorders held at Pace University in New York City, January 1975. It is most appropriate that this material was contributed to a conference honoring the name of the late Dr. Froeschels, who was one of the foremost international authorities on the problem of stuttering and allied disorders of communication. Dr. Froeschels was not only an important contributor to the clinical and experimental research in his field—he also had a great and rare appreciation for the value of historical material, as several of his publications bear witness. He believed, as we do, that an acquaintance with the historical development of a profession or a science is essential for an accurate understanding of present day theory, research, and practice. It provides perspective, stimulates new ideas, promotes clear thinking, and prevents needless duplication of work.

We can do no more in the following pages than touch on a few highlights of the history of stuttering in conjunction with several reprints of early contributions which will be found at the back of this volume. There were, of course, many other contributors than we have space to mention here, but we hope to be able to suggest, in broad outline, the general trend of development, and its connection with the social and intellectual factors of the times and places through which it passed.

R. W. RIEBER
January 1977

DE MORBIS

PVERORVM

TRACTATVS

LOCVPLETISSIMI,

Variàq; doctrina referti non folùm Medicis, verum-
etiam Philofophis magnopere vtiles;

Ex ore Excellentißimi Hieronymi Mercurialis Forolitienfis
Medici clarißimi diligenter excepti, atque
in Libros tres digefti :

Opera Iohannis Chrofczieyoioskij

CVM LICENTIA, ET PRIVILEGIO.

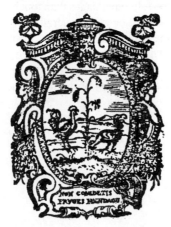

Venetijs, Apud Paulum Meietum Bibliopolam Pat.
M. D. LXXXIII.

We here reproduce for the reader the title page of the *Treatise on the Diseases of Children*
(1583) by Hieronymus Mercurialis. The section on speech defects of this great medical
work of the Renaissance, in a new translation by Jeffrey Wollock, is the opening chapter of
Part II of this volume (see p. 127).

THE HISTORICAL ROOTS OF THE THEORY AND
THERAPY OF STUTTERING

R. W. RIEBER

The John Jay College, City University of New York, 444 West 56th Street, New York 10019

AND

JEFFREY WOLLOCK

Section on the History of Psychiatry and the Behavioral Sciences,
Cornell University Medical College,
925 East 68th Street, New York, NY 10021

The history of the problem of stuttering, one of the best known yet least understood disorders of communication, begins with several brief mentions of *"trauloi"* by Hippocrates (460–377 B.C.). Although we can be sure that this word refers to a speech defect of some kind (it is very likely a generic term that would today be regarded as several distinct defects), its exact meaning is far from clear. Particularly in the books of the *Epidemics,* the passages are quite obscure, as their definitive commentator, Galen (131–ca 200 A.D.), readily admitted. This did not stop him from making some kind of sense of them, however. Since the subsequent history of the subject is largely derived from these Galenic commentaries, at least up to the beginnings of the scientific revolution of the seventeenth century, a few general remarks would be in order.

In the first place it is impossible to understand the earlier history of stuttering unless we realize that no basic distinction was made between stuttering, cluttering, disarthria, functional articulation problems, and even some types of aphasia. Secondly, as a corollary to this, the terminology for these various conditions was anything but precise. We find each of the terms *traulosis, psellismos, blaesitas, balbuties,* and to some extent *mogilalia,* used to describe every one of these conditions, while *ischnophonia,* which very clearly means stuttering in the works of Aristotle, just as clearly describes a weak voice in the works of Galen. Thirdly, the humoral system of medicine, which Galen espoused, and which became the framework of medieval and renaissance medicine, made no diagnostic disjunction between mind and body. For this reason it is somewhat misleading to think in terms of a "humoral physiology" and a "humoral psychology" (useful as these concepts may be in tracing the development of the respective modern disciplines of those names), because no real separation appeared until the humoral system was already in an advanced state of decay.

With the lack of such clear distinctions, the Galenic writings on stuttering at first appear almost totally worthless to the modern investigator. Their meaning emerges only if we realize the great conceptual differences between the Galenic and the modern system.

According to the ancient view, the entire universe originates in four qualities, heat, cold, moisture, and dryness. Out of the combinations of these in pairs arise four elements. Heat and dryness produce fire, heat and moisture produce air, cold and dryness produce earth, cold and moisture produce water.

As man is a microcosm, or miniature of the universe as a whole, these four elements have their equivalents in the human organism, namely, the four *humors,* yellow bile, blood, black bile, and phlegm, which are directly responsible for the condition (or "complexion") of the body and mind. These humors did not exist in a pure state, but were constantly shifting in proportion, depending on the relations of the "six non-natural things" to the organism. The term non-natural refers to circumstances that are not inborn—quality of air, motion and exercise, food and drink, state of excretions, state of passions and affections of the mind, and sleep and dreams. There is nevertheless a *natural* temperament. That is, every individual is born with one of the humors predominating over the others, from which he derives a predominant cast, or temperament, of mind and body.

In the hot and dry temperament, "choleric" or "bilious," an abundance of yellow bile causes the characteristics of fire to predominate. In the hot and moist, or "sanguine" temperament, an abundance of blood causes the characteristics of air to predominate. The cold and dry, "melancholic" has the characteristics of earth, and the "phlegmatic," of water.

We cannot go into the details here of the various casts of voice and speech associated with each temperament. What has been said so far will be enough to demonstrate, however, that the classical concept of speech defects was entirely different from the modern, and followed from the characteristics of the several temperaments. The surviving passages of Galen on speech defects represent not a complete doctrine, but only small fragments of one. It is known that Galen wrote a book on the voice, which may well have contained a more complete statement on speech defects, but as this is one of about 400 treatises of his that have been lost, we have no way of knowing. We can, however, supplement what we have from Galen with further fragmentary insights from Aristotle, particularly Book XI of the *Problems,* and commentaries by later writers who based their own thoughts on the subject almost entirely on these two sources. The extraordinary homogeneity of the basic concepts in medieval and renaissance medicine seems to allow the following attempt at a reconstruction.

The names for the various defects were interchanged so readily because these were not names of clinical entities, like the modern "stuttering" or "cluttering." Rather, they were names for *symptoms,* and a description of the symptoms, no matter how brief, was more important than the particular names given to it. To them the actual disease was not the speech defect, but the humoral imbalance affecting the whole organsim. But in order to know what this was, it was necessary to determine the natural temperament unique to each patient by a thorough examination of every part of the body and an appraisal of the state of mind. "Stuttering" in a phlegmatic person, therefore, had an entirely different etiology from "stuttering" in a choleric person, no matter what names were used. The ancients also recognized the importance of organic speech defects. Those that were not caused by accident or disease were attributed to humoral imbalance in the "original conformation" of the organ.

There still remains considerable ambiguity of course, but that is because within a given temperament, and taking account of the multitude of in-between shadings, the course of development of various speech defects was thought to be the same. Even today we find these symptoms appearing in many combinations with each other. The "distemper" (or imbalance of the normal temperament) was more significant to the ancients than the particular speech defect (see Fig. 1).

Particularly worthy of mention in the transition from Greek to medieval times are the accounts of speech defects given by the Arabic writers Rhazes and Avicenna.

An elaborate example of the renaissance approach to medical problems is found in the section on speech defects in the *Treatises on the Diseases of Children* of Hieronymus Mercurialis (1583) published at Venice in 1583. (See Wollock's new translation of this treatise, p. 127. The great physician of those times was expected to be a great classical scholar as well, because so much of the medical activity consisted of collecting, editing, translating, and harmonizing every statement (in some cases every word) of the ancients on a particular topic. Mercurialis was the first to accomplish this with regard to speech defects. One of our contributors, Dr. Stanley Ainsworth (1957), continues this task of integration at

"Quatuor humores in nostro corpore regnant"

ELEMENTS	PROPERTIES	HUMORS	TEMPERAMENTS
Air	warm and moist	blood	sanguine (hopeful)
Earth	cold and dry	black bile (spleen)	melancholie (sad)
Fire	warm and dry	yellow bile (liver)	choleric (erasible)
Water	cold and moist	Phlegm (brain & lung)	Phlegmatic (apathetic)

Fig. 1

the present time—particularly important in a field with so many rival theories as ours.

One point brought up by Mercurialis is of special interest to us today:

> . . . it seems to me that Aristotle explained this better than anyone else in that passage, *Problems xi. 38,* where, asking why the hesitant of tongue were melancholics, he wrote that all melancholics have quick motions of the imagination, and that [stutterers][1] therefore, since they do have these quick motions, are melancholy as well. He says also, moreover, that [stutterers] have quick motions because, since the instruments of the tongue itself are weak, and cannot exactly follow the concepts of the mind, it happens that the mind's motions always anticipate those of the tongue, and hence the impediment of tongue.

Ideas of this kind seem to appear in every period, including our own, sometimes in the crude form of an "old wives' tale" or parents complaint, but also couched in the prevailing theoretical framework of the various periods. These formulations, despite their unfamiliar language, are all attempts to explain the phenomenon of stuttering by suggesting a failure of synchronization between the processes of thinking and speaking. We will have more to say about this and its relationship to contemporary theory in the conclusion of this paper.

With regard to his treatment, Mercurialis was just as eclectic as he was with his theories. He made a careful diagnosis and attempted to differentiate various communication disorders. Some he attributed to dental problems, others to insufficiency in the capacity of the speech musculature, etc. He treated the symptoms as well as the cause. If he thought the stuttering problem was caused by dryness, he sought to change the conditions of the body by adding moisture. If he attributed the stuttering problem to coldness and humidity, he sought to treat this condition by prescribing warming and drying substances.

Mercurialis also had his own psychotherapeutic technique. He stressed the importance of avoiding fear because he believed that fear aggravated the problem of stuttering by producing a cold condition of the properties in the speech mechanism. He also believed that fear prevented the necessary development of self-confidence and personal accomplishment in the stutterer. To counteract the effects of fear, Mercurialis used what he called trepidation. Mercurialis' notion of trepidation might be interpreted as a special condition of fear analogous to what today is called existential anxiety. Mercurialis felt that this emotion could help the individual to encounter what he feared. Trepidation, therefore, was a kind of psychotherapeutic technique to instill self-confidence and nurture self-accomplishment. He advocated other therapeutic techniques such as vocal exercises, e.g., deep and clear speaking.

Mercurialis advised that men should refrain from excessive lovemaking (but did

---

[1] Mercurialis here uses the word *balbi* (see Translator's Note on p. 127. But it is clear from the original passage of Aristotle, who uses the word *ischnophonoi,* that stutterers are meant.

not apply this to women). He advised against bathing the head of stuttering children, since this would increase the humidity. He advised that bowel movements should be smooth and regular, and that the use of wine should be moderate. With regard to diet he recommended aromatic, salty, and sharp food and advised abstinence from the use of pastries, nuts, and fish. The basic concept was to dry out and warm the entire system. Once all this was accomplished, the body was to be purged.

The age of scientific experimentation was influenced to a great extent by the writings of Sir Francis Bacon. This famous savant was interested in virtually everything, including speech and hearing. But when we look at the following brief passage on stuttering included by Bacon in his *Sylva Sylvarum* of 1627, little more than a generation after Mercurialis, we are not struck by any profound change.

> Divers, we see, doe stut. The Cause, may bee, (in most,) the Refrigeration of the Tongue; Whereby it is lesse apt to move, And therefore wee see, that Naturalls doe generally Stut: And wee see that in those that Stut, if they drinke Wine moderately, they Stut, less, because it heateth: And so we see, that they that Stut, doe Stut more in the first offer to speake, than in Continuance; Because the Tongue is, by Motion, somewhat heated. In some also, it may be, (though rarely,) the Drinesse of the Tongue; which likewise maketh it lesse apt to move, as well as Cold; For it is an Affect that it cometh to some wise and Great Men; As it did unto Moses, who was *Linguae Praepiditae;* And many Stutters we finde are very Cholericke men; Choler Enducing a Driness in the tongue.

Every statement in this passage can be found in the classical writers or in biblical legend. What is not immediately apparent from the passage itself is that the stage was being set for an entirely new approach to scientific inquiry. Where previous writers stressed or relied upon the authority of the ancients, Bacon's plea was for exact observation of natural phenomena. In his *Novum Organum* and *The Advancement of Learning* he set down the axioms that were to form the basis of the scientific method of the present. The most evident indication of this in his short passage is simply the absence of citations, for his intent was to use for authority only what he could observe. In this case it did not lead to any original contribution to the theory of stuttering—except for the vast possibilities opened up by the method.

It fell to the eighteenth century to begin to work out these possibilities to some advantage. The main trends of that century were (1) the rise of nosology, or the classification of diseases, an accomplishment we now take so much for granted that we rarely think of its origins, (2) psychology, which in the eighteenth century sought a new explanation of the faculties and operations of the mind and their relationship to the body, based primarily on the desire to understand the *mechanisms* of phenomena, such as the association of ideas and the exploration of sensory-motor processes, (3) pathological anatomy, stressing the careful observation and description of the diseased state of the body, and (4) pedagogical techniques, spurred by the work of phoneticians and teachers of the deaf.

As nosologists we may mention Boissier de Sauvages (1768) and William Cullen (1775), who carried out not the first, and certainly not the last of many futile attempts to clear up the terminology of communication disorders. They did, however, offer a model of desired achievement along the lines of what Linnaeus accomplished for the biological sciences.

One of the first great classification systems was that of Boissier de Sauvages (1768), who identified clinical entities and classified them according to their similarities. It should be pointed out, however, that de Sauvages went beyond the symptomatology of Felix Platter (1656), and gave a background of etiology, anatomy, and therapeutics. This work did much to call attention to the various disturbances of speech and hearing. De Sauvages' classification of these disturbances was quite ingenious. For instance, under the classification of what he called *dyscinesiae,* he lists the following clinical entities:

1. *Mutitas,* which today is analogous to organic articulatory disorders.

2. *Aphonia,* which is similar to organic disorders that result in the loss of the voice.

3. *Psellismus,* including what we today call disorders of rate and rhythm (stuttering and cluttering), but also various functional articulation defects.

4. *Paraphonia,* an entity similar to defects of vocal quality.

De Sauvages' system was rather static and elementalistic in nature. He went too far in making every minor observable symptom a subtype of the problem he was describing. The interrelationships of many of these classifications were not clearly understood by de Sauvages.

Other classification systems were developed during this period. For example, Cullen (1775) improved upon de Sauvages' system by synthesizing and cutting down upon the number of clinical entities described. However, his classification of speech and hearing disorders was quite similar to de Sauvages in many respects. He used the same four entities under the same general heading *Dyscinesiae.* Cullen classified articulatory disorders not due to organic problems under the clinical entity *Psellismus.* Seven types were described by Cullen under this heading.

The last of the great eighteenth-century nosologists was Erasmus Darwin. In Darwin's *Zoonomia* (1796) we find a remarkable change in the manner of classifying diseases. He attempted a psychophysiological analysis of behavior, describing four distinct powers or faculties acting upon the body. Because Darwin's discussion of speech disorders primarily dealt with the problem of stuttering as a psychological problem, we will discuss it below under the heading of psychology.

The great figure in the field of pathology during the eighteenth century was Giovanni Battista Morgagni (1682–1771). Morgagni stressed the pathological state of the organism, whereas de Sauvages (1768) neglected the pathological state altogether. Morgagni followed a topographic classification system and described in great detail the pathological changes in the patients he studied. In his book, *Seats and Causes of Diseases,* he described many of the well-known speech disorders. His theory of stuttering was based on the assumption that deviations in the hyoid bone were the cause of the majority of cases of stuttering.

Morgagni's theory was formulated on the basis of his autopsy examinations of the larynx of stutterers. (This was contrary to the doctrine expounded by Galen that speech defects and voice defects were quite distinct from one another.) The methodology of post-mortem examination of organs has the disadvantage of excluding all factors not associated with particular diseased organs, and notably, psychological factors. The real advantage was that Morgagni was for the first time actually describing scientific data, but he made the unfortunate mistake of assuming a causal relation between unusual variations in the hyoid bone and the problem of stuttering. This approach, which brought spectacular results with regard to diseases clearly associated with particular organs, was not applicable to speech. For there is no organ of speech; speech is an overlaid function of the entire organism. For a discussion of Morgagni's descriptions of cases of speechlessness associated with apoplexy, head injury, and cerebral disease, see Benton and Joynt (1960).

Let us turn next to a group of eighteenth century philosopher-psychologists known as the *associationists,* so called because most of them wrote much about the "association of ideas," a phrase popularized by John Locke, and were interested in the question of how simple ideas go together to form complex ideas. Their studies thus gravitated toward the problem of how individuals learn. Men such as David Hartley (1749), Moses Mendelssohn (1783), and Erasmus Darwin (1796) were very much interested in speech and language disturbances, as well as the normal development of speech and language in the child.

The associationists tended to describe mental processes in terms of analysis, the law of "contiguity." In this law, the basis of association was the observation that two objects became associated or linked together when they are perceived or thought of simultaneously or in close succession.

Hartley indicated that sensations (internal feelings stimulated by external events) are associated with simple brain states (vibrations), and ideas (internal feelings other than sensations) are also related to simple brain states. It was theorized that these bonds tie with the simple states into complex compounds. In terms of understanding language, Hartley believed that we arrive at an understanding of one another through the power of association, a process whereby simple sounds are associated into a whole, i.e., words, sentences, and so on. Hartley wrote about auditory images as they relate to the development of speech and language in the child. He believed that children learn to speak by repeating the sounds that stimulate the organism to respond. Speech disorders were interpreted in a similar fashion. For instance stuttering, according to Hartley, develops from fear, eagerness, or a violent passion that prevents the child from using his speech mechanism in the correct manner. The result is a confusion that disrupts the vibrations traveling via neural pathways to the peripheral speech mechanism. Since there is disruption in the normal transmission of the vibrations, the individual reiterates again and again until he is successful. Hartley pointed out, however, that in general this problem would not develop until the child is of an age when he can distinguish right from wrong in the pronunciation of speech sounds. He also felt that stuttering may develop from a "defect of memory from passion" and in some cases that it can be learned by imitation. He went on to point out that stuttering tends to spread or to generalize to other words or situations. It is interesting to note that this basic phenomenon is still being explored by learning theorists interested in the problem of stuttering.

As Brett (1921) points out, Hartley had a strong influence on later scientists who studied language disorders:

> As an analysis it is remarkable and clearly prepares the way for the latter work of speech; i.e., the study of aphasia and its cognates. This is not only true in the general sense but can be stated explicitly. For Charcot says *(Lecons du Mardi, I, 362)* that the root of aphasia is in Hartley, who he studied thoroughly.

In the first volume of the first periodical that dealt solely with problems of a psychological nature *(Magazin fur Erfahrungsseelenkunde)*, Spalding wrote a brief article in the form of an introspective report dealing with a transitory sensory motor aphasia. In the same issue of that journal Moses Mendelssohn (1783) wrote a paper giving his interpretation of Spalding's experience, in which he developed a theory of stuttering. Mendelssohn's theory was very similar to other associationist theories of the time. He postulated that if two ideas of varying degrees, A and B, are causally related, this relationship will continue to operate even if the degree of A and B becomes zero. Here Mendelssohn implied an unconscious mechanism beneath the threshold of awareness. Such an acknowledgment of an unconscious mechanism was not unique during the latter part of the eighteenth century (see Whyte, 1962).

The order in which the impact of affective ideas occurs in the individual is an important aspect of Mendelssohn's theory. Like the other associationists, Mendelssohn felt that emotion can disturb this order, and if such emotion or passions do occur and prove to be detrimental to the physiological order involved, stuttering may result.

Darwin was another associationist who utilized this kind of theory in his interpretation of the problem of stuttering. He believed that *motions* affecting the body might result from the following: *irritations* excited by external factors; *sensation* aroused by pleasure or pain; *volition* aroused by desire or aversion; or *associations* that could be linked with other movements. He interpreted all disorders in terms of one or another of these processes and based his classification of diseases upon this frame of reference.

Darwin's hope was that his classification would present a better understanding of the nature of illness or disease. Greatly influenced by Hartley, Darwin classified the problem of stuttering as a disease of volition, developing his theory around the idea that when the stutterer is very much preoccupied with an idea, the corresponding fear of failure is so great that the associations of the muscular motions of articulation become impaired. The stutterer then attempts in vain to gain voluntary control of these broken associations, resulting in a stuttering bloc that may then cause "various distortions of countenance." The cure for stuttering is as follows (Darwin 1796):

> The art of curing this defect is to cause the stammerer to repeat the word, which he finds difficult to speak, eight or ten times with the initial letter, in a strong voice, or with an aspirate before it, as arable or harable; and at length to speak it softly with the initial letter P, parable. This should be practiced for weeks or months upon every word, which the stammerer hesitates in pronouncing. To this should be added much commerce with mankind, in order to acquire a carelessness about the opinions of others.

Pedagogical techniques in the field of stuttering developed in the eighteenth century mainly as an offshoot of the British elocutionary movement, which arose in response to the demand for higher standards in education and in usage of the English language. We will only concern ourselves here with those individuals who approach the movement from a scientific point of view. In an excellent study, Haberman (1954) deals with the overall aspects of this movement.

John Thelwall (1810–1814) is probably the most outstanding figure in the early scientific phase of the movement. His brilliant contributions have been oversimplified, often overlooked, and sometimes distorted. For instance, we cannot agree with Simion's (1954) opinion that the modern approach, (i.e., human being as an organism functional unity), to the speech and hearing handicapped individual developed as a part of the advancements of science during the twentieth century. Nor can we agree with his statement that "It is quite understandable why the early work and public observations, particularly in speech, were largely the province of the physician or physiologist, with explanations of human deviations and deficiencies being sought anatomically and physiologically in terms of the structure or functioning of specific organs." The historical facts do not support these assertions. The writings of Amman (1700, 1893), Van Helmont (1667, 1694), Hartley (1749), Darwin (1796), Thelwall (1810, 1814), Poett (1828), and many others demonstrate a definite humanistic philosophy toward the speech handicapped individual as well as an awareness of the psychological problems involved with the speech and hearing handicapped.

Thelwall (1810) shows great sensitivity and sophistication in his approach to the understanding of speech and hearing disorders. Space does not permit a complete discussion of Thelwall's contribution; however, we should mention that he was aware of the various levels of etiology (predisposing, maintaining, etc.), especially when he discussed stuttering. He was also very much aware of the problem of recognizing mental retardation and differentiating it from emotional disturbances. His *Letter to Henry Cline on Imperfect Development of the Faculties Mental and Moral* (1810) and his *Results of Experience in the Treatment of Cases of Defective Utterance* (1814) are the best examples of his work in speech pathology. In his later work he shows great insight in pointing out how some children with speech disorders will respond better in therapy with a female therapist rather than a male therapist.

As a part of the elocutionary movement, we should mention the work of Sheridan (1762), who was the first as far as we can determine to use the English term "cluttering speech" to refer to the clinical problem of cluttering. We should also mention the work of John Herries (1773), who did much to improve the conditions and attitudes toward speech handicapped individuals.

Historians of science generally consider the renaissance as the beginning of the modern age. The world of the present began to take form particularly toward the early part of the nineteenth century. Increased activity in economic, political, and intellectual spheres gave rise to an atmosphere of change and ferment. Education began to become available to the masses, and the establishment of more schools and universities in all parts of the world under western influence enabled more of the populace to become literate. The industrial revolution in turn served to improve communications among scholars in various parts of the globe. Consequently, more scientific information could be disseminated through books and journals than ever before.

The nineteenth century likewise brought forth greater interest and more diversified points of view regarding the various disorders of communication, and particularly the problem of stuttering.

Jean Marc Gaspard Itard, a renowned French physician, was very much interested in all aspects of communication disorders. His most famous contribution was a book on the so-called "wild boy of Aveyron." On his first major assignment as staff physician of the Institute for the Deaf in Paris, he directed his effort toward the teaching of communication skills, as well as toward a scientific study of the peripheral speech and hearing mechanisms. His treatise on the diseases of the ear is regarded as a major foundation of modern otology. In 1817, he formulated a theory of stuttering in which he attributed the major cause to a generalized deficiency in the nerves, which failed to stimulate proper innovation of the muscles of the larynx and tongue.

The eighteenth-century faculty psychologists had placed their emphasis on the *universality* of the faculties operating the human mind. This harmonized well with one of the dominant themes of the age, the drive toward centralization and large-scale social and political structures, which sought validity in a scientific notion of the "common man" and his capacities.

Toward the end of the century an increased interest in the individual became noticeable as one of the characteristics of a new philosophy—romanticism. A similar shift took place in psychology. Now the study of the faculties centered not on what was common to all men, but on the characteristics unique to each. An early, prominent manifestation of this tendency was the new doctrine of phrenology instituted by Gall.

Gall's system postulated that localized physiological functions of the brain were responsible for the psychological strengths and weaknesses of the individual. These affected the growth of the skull, and could be determined from a careful inventory of its shape. In France, contemporary with Gall, Cabanis was doing much anatomical work to foster the notion of the brain as the organ of thought, from a materialist standpoint. Although phrenology was not materialism in a strict sense, it obviously had a similar thrust, deriving individual psychology from primarily physiological factors. What had formerly been a metaphysical category (i.e., faculty) was now an area of the brain. Phrenology was carried on after Gall's death by his colleague Spurzheim, by the brothers Combe in Edinburgh, and by Charles Caldwell and the Fowlers in the United States.

Once Kant had raised psychology to a supreme position among the intellectual activities of man, subsequent psychological theories tended to invade every area of life, with results often bizarre, but often fruitful. This was certainly true of phrenology.

It was bound to happen that the phrenologist would eventually address himself to the problem of stuttering. And here, almost unnoticed, occurred a "paradigm drift" of great importance. No longer was the focus directed toward the static concept of the pathology of the peripheral speech organ, as in Morgagni; now we find the more dynamic concept of a process instituted by the brain, depending on a language faculty in the brain, and owing its weaknesses to an inadequate faculty of the brain.

All this is exemplified by a paper that Andrew Combe published in the *Phrenological Journal* of 1826.[2] The essence of his theory of stuttering is that a *conflict* of the active faculties gives a plurality rather than a unity of function to the nervous impulse, leading to a conflict in the transmission of energy to the peripheral speech mechanism, which in turn leads to a plurality of action in speaking. This results in "the ineffectual struggle of a small organ of language to keep pace with the workings of larger organs of intellect," *i.e.,* a lack of synchronization between language and thought, a theme that seems to turn up in every age.

Combe identifies nine observational facts in the problem of stuttering, and interprets these facts to support his theory. His approach (and the theory itself) is reminiscent of the work of the late Robert West on organic brain dysfunction in stuttering (West, 1958). Combe also made the point that parents' ill-judged efforts

---

[2]Reprinted in this volume, p. 146.

can cause the very problem they mean to prevent—a position later elaborated by Wendell Johnson in his *diagnostogenic* theory of stuttering. Since stuttering results from interference of the emotions with the will, Combe advocated a therapy combining exercise with moral "treatment," a nineteenth-century predecessor of psychotherapy. These concepts will be explained below.

The first American to write a scientific paper on the problem of stuttering was Edward Warren (1804–1878), a prominent surgeon at Harvard, son of John Collins Warren and grandson of John Warren, both famous surgeons of their day. Warren, although he showed no special leanings toward phrenology, and cited none of the phrenological literature, offered an explanation of stuttering basically compatible with Combe's.

Warren noted that there was no organic defect of the physical speech organs; no difference could be detected between the organs of stutterers and those of normal speakers. Furthermore, he pointed out that the stuttering itself varied greatly in an individual and sometimes disappeared. Here he faces the question, "does stuttering arise then from purely psychological causes?" And he answers in the negative. Stuttering is a very complex disorder, originating in childhood (or even before birth) in a debility of the nervous system, and more specifically, an irregular action of neural impulses. True stuttering appears when this original weakness is aggravated by fear and by the habitual nature of the problem. Therefore, he believed the cause to be both mental and physical.

In detailing the "exciting causes" of stuttering, Warren mentioned one that deserves special notice.

> Persons who are thus susceptible may be so readily carried away by strong feelings, that in the hurry and earnestness to express their ideas, they crowd their words so rapidly upon each other as to produce stammering. They are constantly the subjects of those ardent emotions that are occasional causes of stammering in good speakers. This is not a place for me to discuss the connection between thought and words. Otherwise, I might prove that the time required for the articulation of a single word is sufficient for a long train of thought to pass through the mind. Now, the earnest endeavor to express thoughts as rapidly as they are conceived will produce stammering. This is what we often witness in persons who are stammerers.

In this passage Warren shows clear awareness of something for which we now have much corroborating evidence: that stuttering and cluttering are closely related. Rieber (1975) and Weiss (1964) have even theorized that cluttering often gives rise to stuttering. In actual cases the two cannot be differentiated as completely separate entities; rather, one or the other predominates, but the symptoms overlap. [see a discussion of this in Rieber (1975)]. Once again we encounter our "old wives' tale."

Warren also describes the symptomatology of stutterers, showing an early use of a distinction familiar today, now identified by the terms tonic and clonic stuttering. He was also interested in the personality of the individual stutterer, pointing out that stutterers are usually of "nervous temperament." Although the humoral system had rapidly fallen away with the advent of modern anatomy and physiology, the system of temperaments, as a useful psychological concept, has survived in some form or other right up to the present time. We have already spoken briefly about the ancient doctrine of the four temperaments and its connection with speech pathology. In the meantime considerable modifications had taken place. According to D. H. Jacques,[3] Georg Ernst Stahl first adapted the four temperaments to modern views of physiology and pathology. At a later date Dr. John Gregory added a fifth, which he called the "nervous temperament," while William Cullen, his colleague at the University of Edinburgh, reduced them to only two, the sanguine and the melancholic. Richerand, in this *Elements of Physiology*, considered the melancholic temperament of the ancients, as well as Gregory's nervous temperament, to be diseased rather than normal states.

Until the time of Gregory, insufficient account had been taken of the brain in the process of tempering the constitution. It had played far more of a physiological than a psychological role as an organ that was thought to cool the blood and supply moisture to the head. It did not begin to take its proper place until Gall and Spurzheim modified the system, adopting the nervous temperament of Gregory. Spurzheim's system appears to be the one most used during the nineteenth century. (See Fig. 2, p. 16). He groups the temperaments into *lymphatic* or (phlegmatic), characterized by slowness, weakness of vegetative, affective, and intellectual functions, paleness, fair hair, and roundness of form; *sanguine:* easily affected by external impressions, greater energy than the other temperaments, consistency of flesh, moderate plumpness of parts, animated countenance, light or chestnut hair; *bilious:* strong, marked and decided expression, great general activity and functional energy, black hair, dark complexion, harsh features; and *nervous:* great nervous sensibility, brilliant imagination, highly emotional, quick in perception, desiring novelty and change, fine thin hair, weak muscles.

Two of these temperaments, the lymphatic and the nervous, were considered to be affected by pathology. It was the nervous type, characterized by excessive development of the morbid activity of the nervous system, that Warren identified as the typical stutterer. Warren noted that stuttering seldom continues into adulthood, unless maintained by psychological factors; if it does, moral treatment is required. Andrew Combe, as mentioned above, also advocated this approach. Moral treatment grew out of a new emphasis on feelings and emotion in the philosophy and psychology of late eighteenth and nineteenth century romanticism, and a reaction against the amoral tendencies of rationalism. It emphasized, for example, that a person who was quite rational might nevertheless be suffering from a weak or diseased moral sense. According to this view, heredity produced in such people some kind of defective organization of the personality, producing a disproportionate amount of energy or sensibility that leads to an imbalance

---

[3]*The Temperaments* (New York, 1879), pp. 38–39.

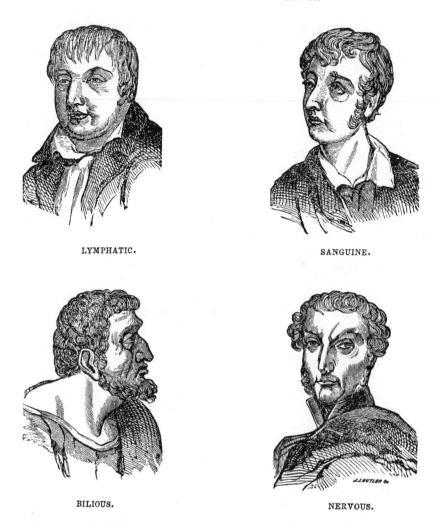

LYMPHATIC.   SANGUINE.

BILIOUS.   NERVOUS.

Fig. 2.   A nineteenth century conception of the four temperaments, from the *American Phrenological Journal*, 1842.

between the passions and the will. "Morality" in this sense pertained to the duty to obey one's conscience in all things, and included correct speech. Through all this echoes one of the watchwords of the age: Kant's "you *can,* because you *must*."

Moral treatment, then, was a therapy to restore this balance between emotion and will. Since the emotion of the stutterer was interfering with his will to speak, it must be replaced by new emotions appropriate to the actions that *ought* to be carried out.

Our next authority, Andrew Comstock (1841), a Philadelphia M.D., was the author of a *System of Elocution, with Special Reference to Gesture, to the Treatment of Stammering and Defective Articulation*. Comstock believed that the cause of stuttering was psychological in most cases, and that the basic problem was the inability of the peripheral mechanism to "obey the commands of the will." A varied treatment, which he called "medico-elocutionary," was required, with the skills of both elocutionist and physician necessary to implement it. Although Comstock did not mention Warren, their positions are compatible. Comstock devised a graduated regimen of exercises for the stutterer, in the belief that these would work, like any other physical therapy, to perfect the various speech behaviors. He gives specific praise to James Rush for his system of elocution, praising him as one of the greatest minds of the century in that field.

The middle of the nineteenth century gave rise to a great deal of additional activity in the field of speech pathology. This was particularly true for the problem of stuttering. The romantic philosophy of this century helped shape the specific scientific developments of the period. The period produced heroic surgical operations (Dieffenbach, 1841), strange secretive treatment procedures (Poett, 1827; Boster, 1827), and unusual mechanical devices [(Bates, 1854)—this and many other devices are described in a paper by Katz, p. 181, of this volume] to permanently cure the problem of stuttering. Social and economic factors, which helped spur the industrial revolution during the nineteenth century, were instrumental in bringing about the invention of the various mechanical devices discussed and illustrated in the Katz paper.

Great significance was attributed to the process of vocalization. At one period this was such an important concept that stuttering was referred to metaphorically as "refusal of the voice." The term "glottal spasms" was often used to specify the exact seat of the problem (Dieffenbach, 1841; Bates, 1854). Wingate (1969) (see also p. 45, this volume) suggests that vocalization, especially as it relates to rhythm, is a crucial factor in understanding and in treating the problem of stuttering. He recommended focusing future research around this approach. One may hope that Wingate finds his approach more fruitful than those of the nineteenth century experts.

Brief mention will be made of Dieffenbach's surgery and Bates' appliance. Dieffenbach (1841), a German surgeon, assumed that stuttering was caused by spasms of the glottis. His treatment consisted of making a horizontal surgical, incision at the root of the tongue. His next step was to make a triangular wedge across the tongue, thereby dividing the lingual muscles. The end result was to eliminate muscular spasms, especially those that occur at the glottis. The Dieffenbach operation was quite popular and allegedly cured a great many stutterers during its brief existence. Dieffenbach was supposed to have operated on over one hundred patients within a year's time. Since most of his colleagues could not duplicate his results, however, the technique was abandoned (see Stevenson, 1968).

Thirteen years later, in the United States, similar enthusiasm was generated by a Mr. Bates, who invented an appliance that he felt would finally eliminate both articulatory and stuttering problems. The Committee of Science and Arts of the Franklin Institute in Philadelphia was so impressed by Mr. Bates' therapeutic instruments that they awarded him a special premium. Bates' instruments resembled a "do-it-yourself therapy kit." For fifteen dollars, anyone could purchase this extraordinary equipment. A special silver tube was used for the curing of articulatory problems. The tube was inserted in the mouth close to the palate, and was designed to overcome problems in the pronunciation of lingual-palatal sounds by providing a continuous flow of air through the oral cavity. The final result was to eliminate the muscular spasm.

A collar-belt was designed to cure the problem of stuttering. It was easily concealed around the neck in a cravat. The collar was securely placed around the neck and was fitted with a special metal plate that was designed to rest upon the thyroid cartilage. A regulator adjusted the desired pressure to be placed on the cartilage. Pressure was applied so that it approximated the thyroid to the artyenoid cartilage.

This counteracted the spasms at the glottal level and produced normal speech. The technique is said to have been extremely popular as well as financially successful. Similar instruments are still for sale today, specially designed to cure the problem of stuttering (see Derazne, 1966); Wohl, 1968). The nineteenth century speech spasm became a powerful lure. Most scientists were attracted to it. Unfortunately, many researchers of this period became so obsessed with the idea of the "spasm" that they hardly progressed beyond it.

The latter part of the nineteenth century gave birth to some of its most dedicated scholars, many of them from Germany. Men such as H. Klencke (1842, 1862), A. Kussmaul (1881), and Albert Gutzman (1887, 1898, 1924) comprised the German schools. James Hunt, Alexander M. Bell, and John Wiley worked out of the British Isles. We have barely broached our subject in this brief outline. A great deal more, in particular, might be said about the latter part of the nineteenth century. But this will have to be left to a future paper.

Throughout this paper we have encountered a number of basic concepts, which seem to be "perennials" in the theory and therapy of stuttering, despite the fact that they may be couched in conceptual frameworks having somewhat different theoretical and philosophical implications.

The first of these is the notion of debility of a particular organ or process. One of the chief remedies proposed for this in all periods has been exercise. In fact all therapy, with the possible exception of drug therapy, includes exercise, e.g., behavior modification, garden-variety psychotherapy, as well as typical speech therapy techniques.

As for pharmaceutical treatment of stuttering, we should note that many topical preparations and purgatives (for humors) were prescribed by Dioscorides, Rhazes,

Avicenna, and others. Such treatments are frequent throughout the renaissance, and Mercurialis included a few in his treatise (p. 127, this volume).[4]

Debility, depending on the frame of reference used, was linked either to superabundance of moisture, as in the humoral writers, to the pathology or defective anatomy of the organ, as in Morgagni, or to a description of the abnormal transmission of vibrations and related associations of ideas, as in Hartley and Darwin. During the nineteenth century, debility was usually mentioned as a cause in connection with the malfunction of a particular organ, such as the tongue, vocal chords, or brain. During the twentieth century the term debility fell somewhat out of fashion, but the concept lingered on in certain quarters, no longer applied to particular organs, however, but to internal systems such as the endocrine, autonomic nervous, central nervous, and metabolic systems. Dysphemia, for example, used by Van Riper (1939) and Green and Wells (1927), was basically a concept of debility. The notion of "delayed myalinization" used by Karlin (1965) is another example.

Our second "perennial" is the concept of conflict. This refers to any two tendencies, or system of tendencies, leading to opposed or divergent actions. The entire humoral system partakes of this element of conflict, which is present in the writings from Aristotle to Mercurialis. Hartley described it in terms of conflicting vibrations and consequent conflicting association of ideas. Darwin described it in terms of internal conflict of the will. The phrenologists of the nineteenth century described stuttering in terms of the conflict of the active faculties, intellect, and language. The twentieth century gave rise to many conflict theories as well. The two most important in this period were the "hemispheric conflict" approach exemplified by Orton (1939) and Travis (1931). This viewpoint stressed the conflict of motor patterns of the two hemispheres of the brain. The other was Sheehan's (1958) theory, which describes stuttering as a double approach-avoidance conflict resulting from a desire to speak and a fear of speaking.

Our final "perennial" is really a variant of the preceding. This is the concept that we have referred to as the "old wives' tale." It appears most frequently today in the intuitive feeling of some parents that their child "thinks faster than he can speak." Technically we would describe this as a dissynchronization between cognitive planning or thinking and speech production or talking. Fully elaborated in a contemporary neuropsychological framework the "old wives' tale" might be explained as follows.

What enables a particular individual, even a stutterer, a clutterer, or aphasic, to engage in what we call "normally fluent behavior"? Obviously, we do not know the full answer to this question. If we did know we probably would be able to

---

[4]For a convenient summary of contemporary views regarding pharmaceutical treatment of speech problems, see Jaffe et al. (1973), pp. 227–228.

discover the many factors that cause stuttering and allied disorders of communication.

Nevertheless, dysfluencies are part and parcel of every day events in the communicative life of an individual. Somewhere along a continuum of fluency behavior, the clinician recognizes a point where a given speaker displays a particular linguistic style that may be characterized by a certain degree of fluency failure. Each individual has his own unique style of communicating. Depending on his perception of this style of language behavior the clinician, or experimenter, correctly or incorrectly, depending on his point of view, diagnoses the behavior of stuttering, cluttering, aphasia, or normal dysfluency. Whatever the final decision may be in terms of diagnosis, one thing becomes clear, namely, that the temporal rate of speech is a key factor in differential diagnosis.

Related to this important factor of temporal rate are several other variables. These are (1) degree of intelligibility, (2) vocalic and intervocalic segments, and (3) pause time and phonation time. It is possible that from the above measures one may arrive at an estimate of a specific degree of fluency in a given speaker. In order for us to accomplish this task we must focus on both the macroscopic and microscopic levels of the communicative process. This would include data that deal with the following sublevels: (1) semantic, (2) lexical, (3) morpheme, (4) phoneme, and (5) motor-control. Once these data are collected they can be utilized, both clinically and experimentally, by relating them to the basic time dimension in communication.

Language is the manifestation of an inner event that we experience as a Gestalt. On the other hand, at another level, it is specific spatiotemporal behavior, which can be analyzed into its component parts.

The failure to find the proper homeostatic union between the whole and the sum of the parts could result in specific ''abnormal'' or disordered spatiotemporal linguistic adjustments. If this assumption is correct, it is then possible that a failure of the necessary spatiotemporal coordination between any of Fry's (1969) levels (semantic, lexical, morpheme, phoneme, or motor-control) could be instrumental in bringing about stuttering, cluttering, or aphasia. The more quickly you are impelled to program your spatiotemporal adjustments, the more likely you are to clutter your words. On the other hand, the more compelled, i.e., ego-alien, you are about programming in speech, the more likely you are to stutter or hesitate on a word. In this sense both stuttering and cluttering appear to be opposite poles of a single dimension of fluency failure. The swing of the pendulum to either extreme of the continuum may account for the clinical observations that clutterers may develop stuttering symptoms during therapy and that stuttering and cluttering are often symptoms found in the same individual. To put it another way, one might say that a stutterer, as a speaker, attempts to proceed so hastily that he does not reach his destination in time, whereas the clutterer attempts to go so fast that he reaches his destination ahead of time. Neither of them are ''on time'' or ''in time,'' as it were, with the normal psychophysiological processes. The same metaphor can be applied to compare the Broca aphasic with the jargon (Wernicke's) aphasic. It is not at all uncommon to find quasistuttering or stuttering-like behavior in aphasic patients.

This observation suggests several questions: (1) What aspects of neuropsychological brain function can account for the facts about the problem of stuttering? (2) How might these neuropsychological processes be related to the individual's psychological reactions and/or to the attention he may exhibit to his own communicative behavior?

In answer to the above questions we would like to suggest the following theoretical position.[5] The human brain can be understood as having certain biologically interdependent neurophysiological mechanisms. The first of these mechanisms might be referred to as a temporal ordering process and the second as a spatial ordering process. The temporal function provides an overall time frame for a given utterance such as a syllable, word, or sentence, etc. The spatial or serial or sound production provides the appropriate sequence of motor events, i.e., articulation within a given time frame during the communicative act. The abovementioned interdependent processes interact with one another in order to achieve the complex event of producing the smooth flow of speech during the communicative act. This event is often referred to as fluency or fluent speech. If we assume that the above mentioned functions may be malfunctioning or out of phase with one another, the most likely result would be a specific kind or class of fluency failure. The manner in which fluency failure manifests itself would also be dependent on the organisms's reaction to or anticipation of this failure in fluency. The quality of attention and/or expectation of the organism's response to this fluency failure would be a crucial determinant of the type of behavior exhibited. When attention and/or expectation is shifted from its appropriate operation of cognitive planning to the operation of phonetic production, this tends to deautomotize the communicative behavior. The result is usually a symptom such as stuttering or cluttering and perhaps certain types of aphasia. Rieber et al. (1976) have shown that fluency failure in stutterers and clutterers is more than likely to occur on the first sound of a word rather than at any other point. Furthermore, it is more likely to occur in a polysyllabic rather than a monosyllabic word. The reason for this phenomenon may be due to the relatively higher order of operational complexity involved in both the temporal and serial ordering of polysyllabic utterances. It should also be noted that not only are monosyllabic words much simpler to program in time and space, but they are also the most frequently used words in spoken and written English.

---

[5]This theoretical model will be elaborated upon in a chapter that will appear in a book edited by R. W. Rieber and D. Aaronson. *Psycholinguistic Research,* to be published late 1977 (L.E.A., New York).

We have discussed a few of the more important books and theories that reflect the diversity that has been manifested in the history of stuttering. Authorities have differed in their definitions of the subject matter, both in selection of problems for study as well as methods for theoretical conceptualization. But these differences have stimulated the intensity and scope of scientific inquiry. They have insured the growth and development of scientific knowledge by providing, as it were, a homeostatic system of checks and balances. However, the full value of this inheritance can be realized only when it comes within the scope of the contemporary quest for knowledge.

References

Amman, J. C. *Dissertatio de loquela*. Amsterdam: Walters, 1700.

Amman, J.C. *A dissertation on speech* (reprint of the 1893 edition) (R. W. Rieber, Ed.), Amsterdam: North-Holland Publishing Co.

Ainsworth, S. Methods for integrating theories of stuttering. In L. Travis (Ed.), *Handbook of speech pathology*. New York: Appleton-Century-Crofts, 1971, p. 1095.

Aristotle. *Aristotle's complete masterpiece* (23rd ed.). London, 1749.

Barbara, D. A. *Stuttering—a Psychodynamic approach*. New York: Julian Press, 1954.

Bastian, H. C. *Aphasia and other speech defects*. London, 1898.

Bates, R. Report of the Committee of Science and Arts. J. Franklin Institute, Philadelphia, 1854.

Benton, A. L., Joynt, R. J. Early descriptions of aphasia. *Arch. Neurol.*, 1960, **3**.

Blume, F. *Neueste-heilmethode des stotteruebels* (Newest Method to Cure Stuttering). Berlin, 1844.

Bormann, E. G. Ephphatha or some advice to stammerers. *J. Speech Hearing Res.*, 1969, **12**, No. 3.

Brett, G. S. *A history of psychology*, Vol. 2. London: George Allen and Unwin, 1921, pp. 283–284.

Broca, P. Sur le siege de la faculte du language (the seat of the faculty to speak). *Bull. Soc. Anat.*, 1861.

Broster, J. *The rise and progress of the brosterian system*. London, 1827.

Comstock, A. *System of elocution, with special reference to gestures to the treatment of stammering and defective articulation*. *Philadlephia, 1841*.

Cullen, W. Synopsis nosologiae methodicae. Amsterdam: Toures, 1775.

Darwin, E. *Zoonomia, or the laws of organic life*. London: Johnson, 1796.

Derazne, J. Speech pathology in the U.S.S.R. In R. W. Rieber and R. S. Brubaker (Eds.), *Speech pathology*. Amsterdam: North-Holland Publishing Co., 1966.

Dieffenbach, J. F. Memoir on the Radical Cure of Stuttering by a Surgical Operation. London, 1841.

Dorrance, G. M. *The operative story of cleft palate*. Philadelphia: W. B. Saunders Co., 1933.

Eldridge, M. *A history of the treatment of speech disorders*. London: Livingstone, 1968.

Eliasberg, W. G. A contribution to the pre-history of aphasia. *J. Hist. Med.*, 1950, **5**, (1), 96.

Franck, H. *Praxeos medicae universae praecepta* (Prescriptions in medical practice). Leipzig, 1823.

Fry, D. B. The linguistic evidence of speech errors. *Bruno Studies in English*, 1969, **8**, 69–74.

Green, J. S., Wells, E. J. *The cause and cure of speech disorders*. Macmillan: New York, 1927.

Gutzmann, A. *Das stottern* (Stuttering). Berlin: Rosenheim, 1887.

Gutzmann, H. Sr. *Das stottern* (Stuttering). Berlin: Rosenheim, 1898.

Gutzmann, H. Sr. *Sprachheilkunde* (Logopedics) (3rd ed.). Berlin: Fishers, 1924.

Haberman, F. W. English sources of American elocution. In K. R. Wallace (Ed.), *History of speech education in America*. New York: Appleton-Century-Crofts, 1954.

Hartley, D. *Observations on man*. London: S. Richardson, 1749.

Herries, J. *Treatise on the elements of speech*. London: Edward Charles Dilly, 1773.

Holder, W. An account of an experiment concerning deafness. *Phil. Trans. R. Soc.* 1668, 667, **35**, (also found in the appendix of Holder's *Elements of speech*. London: J. Martyn, 1669).

Hoepfner, T. *Stottern als Assoziative Aperatrachtungweise. z. Pathopsychol.*, 1912, 448–453.

Jaffe, J. Anderson, S.W., Rieber, R. W. Research and clinical approaches to disorders of speecn rate. *J. Commun. Dis.*, 1973.

Kaiser, L. *Manual of phonetics*. Amsterdam: North-Holland PUbl. Co., 1957.

Karlin, I.W. et al. *Development and disorders of speech in childhood*. Springfield, Ill.: C. C. Thomas, 1965.

Klencke, H. *Untersuchungen und Erfahrungen in der Anatome, Physiologie, Mikrologie* (Research and experiences in anatomy, etc.). Leipzig: Kollman, 1842.

Klencke, H. *Heilung des Stotterns* (Cure of stuttering). Leipzig: E. Kollman, 1862.

Kussmaul, A. *Die Storungen der Sprache* (The impediments of speech) (4th ed.). Leipzig: F. C. W. Vogel, 1881.

McCormac, H. *The cause and cure of hesitation of speech or stammering*. London, 1828.

Mendelssohn, M. Psychologische Betrachtungen auf Veranlassung einer von Spalding, *Mag. Erfahrungsseelenkunde, 1783*, **1**, Part 3 (Berlin) 1783.

Mercurialis, H. *De morbis puerorum*. Venice: Paulus Meletus, 1583.

Morgagni, G. B. The Seat and Causes of Disease, Book I. Letter XIV, London, 1769.

Orton, S. *Reading, writing, and speech problems in children*. New York: Norton, 1939.

Platter, F. *Praxis medicae*. Basil: Konis, 1656.

Poett, J. Sr. *Observations on psellismus, or stammering, with accompanying cases of cure*. Dublin: Joseph Blundell, 1828.

Rieber, R. W. A study in psycholinguistics and communication disorders. *Linguist. Intern. Rev.*, 1975, **160**, 33–70.

Rieber, R. W., Froeschels, E. An historical review of the European literature in speech pathology. In R. W. Rieber and R. S. Brubaker (Eds.), *Speech pathology*. Amsterdam: North Holland, 1966.

Rieber, R. W., et al. Neuropsychological aspects of stuttering and cluttering. In R. W. Rieber (Ed.), *The neuropsychology of language*. New York: Plenum Publishing Co., 1976.

Riverius, L. *The practice of physic in seventeen several books* (translated by N. Culpeper). London: F. Streater, Book 5, Chap. 4, 1668, pp. 127–128.

de Sauvages, F. B. *Nosologia methodica*, Vol. I. Amsterdam: Tournes, 1768.

Schulthess, R. *Das Stammeln und Stottern*. Zurich, 1930.

Sheehan, J. G. Theory and treatment of stuttering as an approach avoidance conflict. *J. Psychol.*, 1953, **56**, 27–49.

Sheridan, T. *A course of lectures of elocution*. London: W. Strahan, A. Millar, 1762.

Simon, C. T. The development of education in speech and hearing to 1920. In K. R. Wallace (Ed.), *History of speech education in America*. New York: Appleton-Century-Crofts, 1954.

Sokolowsky, R. Beziehungen der Sprach—und Stimmleilkunde zur Operativen Laryngologie (Relationship of Logopedics and Phoniatrics to Surgical Laryngo-Rhinology). 3rd Meeting of the Germany Society for Logopedics, Leipzig, 1931.

Stevenson, L. G. The surgery of stammering: a forgotten enthusiasm of the nineteenth century. *Bull. Hist. Med.*, 1968, **42**, 527–554.

Thelwall, J. *A letter to Henry Cline, Esq. on imperfect development of the faculties mental and moral as well as constitutional and organic and on the treatment of impediments of speech*. London: Richard Taylor and Co., 1810.

Thelwall, J. *Results of experience in the treatment of cases of defective utterance, from deficiencies in the roof of the mouth and other mal-conformations of the organs of speech. London: J. McCreery, 1814.*

Travis, L. (Ed.). *Handbook of speech pathology*. New York: Appleton-Century-Crofts, 1957.

Travis, L. *Speech pathology*. New York: Appleton, Century-Crofts, 1931.

Van Helmont, F. M. *Alphabeti vere naturalis Hebraici*. Abrahami Lichtenthaler, Sulzbaci, 1667.

Van Helmont, F. M. *The spirit of diseases or diseases from the spirit*. London.

Van Helmont, F. M. *The spirit of diseases: layed open in some observations concerning man and his diseases*. London: Sarah Howkins, 1694.

Van Riper, C. *Speech correction. Principles and methods*. New York: Prentice-Hall, 1939.

Wallace, K. R. et al. *History of speech education in America*. New York: Appleton-Century-Crofts, 1954.

Watson, J. *Instruction of deaf and dumb*. London, 1809.

Weiss, D. A. *Cluttering*. Englewood Cliffs, N.J.: Prentice-Hall, 1964.

West, R. W. An agnostic speculation about stuttering. In J. Eisenson (Ed.), *Stuttering, a symposium*. New York: Harper, 1958.

Whyte, L. L. *The unconscious before Freud*. New York: Doubleday, 1962.

Wingate, M. E. Sound and pattern in artificial fluency. *J. Speech Hearing Res.*, **12**, 1969, No. 4.

Wohl, M. T. The electronic metronome—an evaluative study. *British J. Dis. Commun.*, 1968, **3**, No. 1.

Wright, J. *Impediments of speech. Three letters to Sir Charles Bell on the causes and cure of stuttering*. London: Whittaker & Co., 1839.

AUTHENTICITY AND CREATIVITY IN STUTTERING THEORY AND THERAPY

ALBERT T. MURPHY

Special Education Department, Boston University, Boston, Massachusetts 02215

For some years I was an instructor in a program of training young psychiatrists to become Professors of Psychiatry. Once, during an initial meeting with several trainees, one of them asked me if I had been in military service. I replied that I had been a Marine Corps pilot, adding later under questioning that I had indeed flown fighter planes and dive-bombers. My questioner was appalled, asking how it felt to be a warmonger of an elitist, chauvinist group trained to kill, and further asking in her pique if I had participated that week with the hard-hats against the anti-war demonstrators. I was taken aback, my feelings a mixture of incredulity, disappointment, and some anger. I replied that I was amazed that a psychiatrist would pigeon-hole a person, especially in a negative sense, on the basis of a characteristic or condition obtaining 25 years before. The more so with no knowledge of what had happened in that person's life in the subsequent quarter century. I asked if she would so sweepingly evaluate and judge the *present* functioning of one of her patients on the basis of something that was a part of that individual's life 25 years before, and with this we were able to move into a discussion that had professional learning potential.

Not only for her I thought, but of course, for myself as well.

For the incident initiated a particular stream of consciousness in my mind. Many lives were sacrificed in the war, and I very nearly sacrificed my own. For what purpose? It was not because of a patriotism that was only nationalism and it was not because of any deeply held feelings I had for the enemy. As the late Sir Herbert Read once stated, "I was caught by the war, like a young animal that had sprung some trap, and I went into it . . . without enthusiasm of any kind except (the) vague desire (of a 17 year old) for adventure and for an ordeal that would test my courage." Those vague desires were soon quieted by the crude horrors of the actual experience. These were endured to the end, but long before the end I had lost the adolescent enthusiasm that gave some glamour to the early days of wartime training and traveling. As the war rumbled on and thousands were being butchered, I acquired a deep distrust and some hatred for all those who, through their slogans and other propoganda devices, were justifying the war. I did not then have the necessary experience or maturity to see through this fiction. And I continued to fight, as did most, for the simple reason that I could not desert my comrades, and

25

secondarily, but perhaps primarily, because I could not bear to be thought a coward.

In such ways are ideals lost—yet also gained. From the idea of mutually *destructive* relationships—but through the medium of learning about the essential goodness of persons, the fidelity of one person to another, especially in circumstances of common danger, the fidelity of all members of a group as a whole—one can move to the idea of mutually *nurturant* relationships. These are relationships that do not kill or destroy but which exist in purpose to *enhance* or *add* life to life. Among these human relationships are those we call therapy.

Professional Relationships and Assumptions

To be in fruitful relationship is to be in communication in the finest sense. Whatever interferes with communication in this mutually enhancing way constitutes an impairment. Stuttering is one of these impairments. In my own case, an early interest in languages combined with the idea of dysfunctional communication had brought me to the door of Samuel Dowse Robbins of Boston. Himself a stutterer, in addition to being a former President and Secretary for many years of the American Speech and Hearing Association, Sam Robbins had, in addition to the stuttering, the additional handicaps of a remarkable overbite and visual agnosia. I liked him immediately and we developed a close friendship. After my studying stuttering from Robbins' heavy neurophysiological perspective, he recommended that my graduate training occur with any one of three individuals, each of whom he admired greatly: Wendell Johnson, Lee Travis, or Charles Van Riper. Having lived in Los Angeles earlier, I joined Dr. Travis at the University of Southern California. I have never regretted that. And I was lucky enough later to get to know both Johnson and Van Riper as co-workers and friends and to be nurtured by their warmth and brilliance. All of these men are greatly revered.

I have also had opportunities to be with and be affected by Kurt Goldstein, Carl Rogers, Gordon Allport, and Abraham Maslow, by many colleagues and students, and by many, many persons who stutter. Out of such soils and others arises one's conception of stuttering. One views the behavior wholistically or atomistically, behavioristically or phenomenologically; one views the stuttering person as *person* in the large sense, or through the lens of stuttering as target behavior *or* as symptom, as a problem or as an *experience* to be entered into.

And one makes *assumptions* about stuttering and its treatment. Sometimes they are consciously made, other times unconsciously. The effective clinician wishes to be aware of *all* assumptions as critical determinants in the kinds of relationships one develops. Considering the clinician as the most critical instrument of the process, one of our main responsibilities is to increase our reliability and validity, become consciously aware of the assumptions we make, and carefully consider their implications. Let us name just two typical assumptions. Whether or not a clinician accepts them, it would seem, could make a considerable difference in the way he works, his manner of implementing methods, the goals he sets, and his total view of the stuttering process. Assumption one: a stuttering disorder is not simply behavior existing *en vacuo* but behavior that functions for and because of various motivations and purposes. To make this assumption, for example, would cause one to focus at least as much on *why* the child behaves as he does on *what* he is doing. Implications for the kinds of interventions exercised are considerable. Assumption two: what happens to the stuttering disorder affects *total* behavior and vice versa. In making this assumption the clinician would tend to focus more on total programming than on an isolated bit of behavior as can sometimes be the case. The assumption implies that it is impossible to understand, much less detach, the stuttering disorder from one's feelings.

A deep concern with the persons in the process, deeper than even the important concern of method or technique, would include the constant process of self-evaluation, including the evaluation of *assumptions* one makes as critical determinants of methodological efficacy.

Conceptions and Creativity in Stuttering

Could we say that one might have a *poetic* conception of stuttering and therapy? Most conceptions are rational ones—of course, they have value. Is there a place for a poetic image? It would be related not merely to *describing* and *analyzing* behavior, but more to actually *experiencing* the stuttering and the stutterer —experiencing as a way toward conceptualizing it, feeling about it, a way of being or behaving within it, a way of sensing it and acting upon it, a way of being receptive to it. Is it absurd to think of stuttering or of authentic speaking in the framework of poetry? E.E. Cummings once said that "poetry is feeling—not knowing or believing or thinking. Expressing nobody but yourself in words. Whenever you think, or believe, you're a lot of other people, but the moment you feel, you're nobody but yourself. Expressing nobody but yourself is the most wonderful life on earth." Apply this to the stutterer. Apply it to the clinician.

Improvement in stuttering—in the sense of total functioning—is a *creative* event. I regard improvement as a movement from communicative insecurity toward increased humanness and communicative actualization. To grow is to create onself. In person-oriented stuttering therapy both stutterer and clinician invent themselves—each grows by *choosing,* by taking responsibility, becoming free to risk, in not simply being safe. Again apply this to the stutterer. Apply it to the clinician. The case is stated in a lovely way on an ancient tablet on the coast of Greece:

"A shipwrecked sailor buried on this coast
Bids you set sail
Full many a bark, when we were lost,
Weathered the gail."

I envision my work at its best as a process of creating self through a helping relationship with others. This may sound selfish, in the worst sense, but I mean it as growth oriented self-interest in the best sense, an interest in self-improvement that could lead to more productive functioning with others.

Finally, our conception of stuttering varies, too, with the language we use to express our conceptions. Allport thought that clinicians whose theoretical spectacles disclosed a merely *reactive* being were likely to think of their client in terms of past conditioning and potential reconditioning. The vocabulary emanating from this type of postulate is replete with terms like *reaction, response, reinforcement, reflex, respondent,* all sorts of *re*compounds. The reference is backward. What has been is more important than what will be. Terms such as *proaction, progress,* and *production* are characteristically lacking. I have heard Allport say that one would think that the client seated opposite would *protest,* for the language of response negates the subject's immediate certainty that his life lies in the future.

Perhaps, too, as I wrote over a decade ago, we should cite the distinction between semantic and poetic meaning as applied to stuttering theories and therapies. Semantic meaning refers to the neutral naming of a person or process without affective overtones. Poetic meanings metaphorically orient the individual toward others in a motivational, attitudinal, emotional way. While the semantic plane may be more necessary in research and theoretical operations, the working clinician probably will be more effective through at least partial allegiance to the poetic plane.

The questions one might have about therapy would derive from such perspectives as we have just discussed. Most are actually to some degree explicitly suggested by one's conceptions and assumptions about stuttering. I shall not try to state the more obvious ones. Rather, we might ask ourselves additional questions, such as: Is my therapy autobiographical or is it fiction? Do I "ring true"? Do I do what I think I *ought* to do, or what I deeply believe I want to do? Apply these to the clinician. But apply them to the stutterer, also.

If there is one truth about stuttering therapy, I believe it is simply this: Our persons are more important than our techniques. Some clinicians are by nature forcefully directive; others are quite, soft-spoken individuals capable of deep empathy and devoted persistence. All may help stuttering people, regardless of therapy or techniques pursued. And sometimes fail. Methods or materials used in therapy remain insignificant until touched by a spark, the individual clinician's healthy uniquenesses, which elevate them beyond the commonplace. Regardless of approach, one's attitude concerning the personal dimensions of the encounter called therapy, one's blend of thinking, feeling, and doing, even one's way of life deeply affect both the nature of the interaction and its degree of success, be it objectively or subjectively defined. Such behavior can constitute the advocacy of a certain clinical orientation or mood, a form of attitude toward action appropriate with humans who stutter.

Personology and Authenticity

Therapy to be most effective must be authentically *dialogic*. Martin Buber in many of his writings distinguished among three types of dialogue, which I have adapted and found useful in understanding and working with stutterers. *Technical dialogue* is prompted by the need of objective understanding; it makes no pretense of relating to the other in a fully human sense. The primary concern is with the *techniques* of communication (there are persons who speak fluently and with proper articulation but who say little of real content or feeling). The purpose of technical dialogue is frequently to persuade or to convince others of a particular point of view.

In the second form, *monologue disguised as dialogue,* the clinician and stutterer are together in space but may appear to speak in strangely convoluted or circuitous ways. The stutterer in group therapy who does not actively listen to others but only wishes to monopolize speaking time is also representative. The clinician in staff meeting may act similarly. Such persons, as T.S. Eliot has stated, "put on a face to meet the faces that they meet." They are *seeming* persons rather than being, much less becoming persons.

In the third form, *genuine dialogue,* both stutterers and clinicians open themselves to the otherness of their coparticipants. The other persons are kept in mind in their present and particular being and are attended to with the intention of establishing a living mutual relationship. Authentic dialogue may be verbal or silent, and it does not always mean love; it may mean anger. But it is direct, honest, and personal and confirms the humanness of the other even while opposing or differing from him. One can enter genuine dialogue to the extent that one is a real person.

The Ghosts in the Machine

Of course, in stuttering therapy, the purported *cure* must be at least as persuasive as the *stuttering*. This is the case regardless of therapy approach, that is, whether or not the stutterer is seen as a reactive being (positivism, behaviorism, "scientific" approaches), as a reactive being in depth (psychoanalysis, psychodynamic views), or seen as being in the process of becoming (existential psychology, organismic frameworks, third-force psychology, or humanism).

In stuttering, the clinical world has not infrequently been one of common sense in principle and procedure, of a concern with psychodynamics, of trial and error thinking and action, of intuition or hunches, and of focus on interpersonal relationships. It has been a world in which a number of different approaches from different professional disciplines have been used. It is easy to see why the strict behaviorist, with allegiance usually only to publically observable behavior, balks at some clinicians' attention to the symbolic, the illogical, or to the total unity of a situation. For the behaviorist these things cannot be controlled or objectively measured. But some clinicians regard stutterers not simply as reactors but as active originating agents. It is little wonder that behaviorists could refer to such mentalisms as "the ghosts in the machine," although behavior modification procedures are being related more and more to the realm of private experience.

Those who are open to the behavioral approach recognize the similarities with older procedures; they also realize that the new approach has resulted in a systematization of practices that were formerly executed in a less scientific, less experimentally productive, or less testable manner. Of course scientific rigor does not ensure practical application. Furthermore, behavioral programs always stand in danger of choosing trivial goals, because it is the trivial goals that can be most readily translated into testable, operational statements.

We have, however, greeted the new behavioral techniques with considerable enthusiasm. Our profession has always been eager for new sources of assistance, and this is particularly true with regard to stuttering, which has frustrated us from the beginning. We must be careful that our eagerness for assistance does not lead to a premature and perhaps faulty application of behavioral methods. Clinicians who work with large numbers or groups of stutterers may need to be reminded that most reports on behavioral techniques have come largely from laboratory settings and were derived primarily from experiments with single subjects. As a result, to apply these procedures to groups of stutterers or to stutterers in complex social settings, such as classrooms, requires caution.

Clinicians who are enthusiastic about these new techniques usually realize that their belief in the goodness of the approach may, in itself, produce positive therapeutic results. And a doubting Thomas may recall Doestoievsky having his "underground man" state that "the whole meaning of human life can be summed up in the one statement that man only exists for the purpose of proving to himself every minute that he is a man and not an organ-stop"—a subject and not an object.

The impact of Freud's thought, on the other hand, has been due far less to the instrumentalities he provided than to the changed conception of ourselves that he inspired. Changing the stutterer's conception of himself for the good may be of far greater significance than his implementation of technique. Therefore, some clinicians believe that all changes in functioning involve the total organism because the organism functions as a totality; they stress the importance of context uniqueness of any event; they stress the importance of the interdependence of structure and function; they regard motive forces as originating from within the person; they view as critical the person's future orientation (hope or anticipation of what he can become). Such persons will resist the change in clinician functioning wished for by technologically oriented clinicians. It will be at this point that materials or methods usage will encounter or blend with the individual psychology of clinicians and stutterers.

The coming together of technology and the unique individual should not be an encounter, but a working together. If there is a quarrel, let it be, as Frost said, "a lover's quarrel" with as equal an emphasis on "lover" as on "quarrel." "Who will save us," said William Faulkner, "but the scientist and the humanitarian. Yes, the humanitarian in science, and the scientist in the humanity of man."

The creative communicative mood is inconsistent with any attitude that derogates a therapy philosophy or structure that differs from one's own. But one can be considerately critical. Just as we tolerate and respect the various life styles of our clients, we must also respect the various professional lifestyles of other clinicians, especially since the whole truth about stuttering is not yet known. Nearly a century ago, William James made the point that "Even prisons and sickrooms have their special revelations. It is enough to ask each of us that he should be faithful to his own opportunities and make the most of his own blessings, without presuming to regulate the rest of the vast field."

Neglected Components in Stuttering Therapy

A final consideration of therapy will be related to several of its neglected dimensions or components. What is not written about in the mountain of material dedicated to stuttering may turn out to be the most crucial of all, regardless of the basic type of therapy. I am suggesting that the degrees and forms of *hope, faith, love, trust,* and *courage* are among these neglected considerations in stuttering. Full discussions of each are impossible here, but I feel compelled to comment on several, if only briefly.

Faith, for example, is future-oriented. To have faith at all implies a belief in the possibility that something desired can occur. Many of the problems experienced by stutterers derive from past unpleasant experiences, the effects of which persist into and affect their view of the present. Other problems flow from what I term an overemphasis on present-orientation, an inclination to do whatever seems right or efficacious here-and-now, but in the absence of an over-arching perspective that includes past, present, and future, and that denies the value of none of them. Not least important is the degree to which the stutterer has faith in his own capacity to become something more than he now is, in terms of speaking, or in terms of total life functioning. It is quite remarkable in a person who has failed to speak fluently perhaps thousands of times to see him try yet again. The trying must be related to a faith in a possibility, just as a lack of trying may be related to a lack of faith in a possibility. The faith to go beyond such hurt must include a faith in one's ability to learn from experience and to be attracted to the growth possibilities in the relationship, the possibility, I would say, of creating self in relationship with others. Faith's way of being and becoming in the stutterer–clinician relationship is to move with increasing confidence into the risky known and the even more dangerous unknown.

Trust clearly is related to faith. Trusting the other is to let go; it includes an element of risk and a leap into the unknown, both of which take courage. The parent or the clinician may show a lack of trust by trying to squeeze the "helped one" into a mold, or even, perhaps, by caring too much, or overprotecting. Trust mistrusts indoctrination. Indoctrination may emanate from different viewpoints. But indoctrination serves most to satisfy the indoctrinator's needs, not the needs of the one to be helped.

And what of *hope?* It is amazing, given its importance in life, that such a paucity of concern has been demonstrated for this experience in the literature on stuttering individuals. Certainly, success with parents and children varies as hope varies within their individual and combined experiences. The goal in therapy is to work together to come to see that hope is possible, that it can be made real through efficient planning and the tapping of previously unrealized potentials. Hope is not easily achievable in isolation. The creative clinician works to have the participants leave their isolation by engaging them in dialogue, both verbal and nonverbal. He sees that hope must be differentiated from fantasy. He needs to come to see that authentic hope imagines real things, things that have at least some possibility of coming true. Hope must be imagined, and this imagining succeeds best in dialogue. One imagines with. Therapy is often for me a process of imagining with the parents or the stutterer, then going on together in the quest to achieve that which has been imagined.

Creative therapy takes such components into consideration. It tries to point up the strengths and possibilities of the present; it stresses assets more than pathologies in parents or child. It also tries to stir a sense of what is possible in a way that enlarges the goodness of the present in relation to an attainable future —for example, the setting up of realistic goals and the growth experience of working together to reach them. It will take deep support from others and courage from within oneself to try new ways, break fixed belief systems, go beyond safety and nondevelopmental security, to take the risks involved in creative insecurity. To hope is to come to believe, as William James long ago said, that the "pull of the future is as real as the push from behind."

Personal Needs of Clinicians

There are dangers in being a clinician. There is, for instance, the danger of being wanted badly. We can easily be lured into believing that if so many people wish for our services, then surely we have something of great value to give. Of course, we do not always. Then there is the danger of our own insecurities, being manifested most resoundingly in 1975 by the expressions by speech clinicians of apprehension or jealousy concerning the burgeoning domain of learning disorders. Insecurities in stuttering work are reflected by such behaviors as rigid adherence to set methods, chronic belittlement of the views of others, or defensive resistance to working with stutterers having certain characteristics ("too old," "too severe," etc.). We have long recognized the range of styles represented in our profession. Fifteen years ago I wrote about paternal or maternal clinicians who derive satisfaction from a temporary relation as a parent-substitute; sociable, warmly human clinicians who enjoy the opportunity for sustained contact with a variety of personalities; protective clinicians who, projecting upon their clients their own frustrations, try to make them happy; detached clinicians who enjoy as spectators the panorama of experience revealed by stutterers; those who have need to control the lives of others, whatever their theoretical positions. The personal needs of clinicians deserve more attention than we have given them. One could make a good case for the statement that Al Murphy has needed stutterers at least as much as those stutterers who have felt need of him; hopefully, those needs have been increasingly mature ones.

Of course, rather than taking the personal characteristics of the clinician into greater account in the total process of stuttering therapy it is easier simply to focus on more specific, more manipulable behavior over which we can feel a sense of control and, thus, comfort. This is true whether the behavior selected be an apparently simple speech deviation such as the substitution of one sound for another, a difficulty in correctly linking appropriate sound with specific letter, or any simple, easily understood technique for dealing with such behaviors. It is simpler, but neither necessarily wiser nor even sufficiently helpful. The need to know precisely what we are doing, reflected in avoidance of departure from fixed idea or technique, can constitute a danger if it leads to suspiciousness of innovation or of creative thought. Alfred North Whitehead might have termed it the "fallacy of misplaced concreteness." Similarly, I have referred to a clinically creative act as "the truth of well-placed abstractness."

On the other hand, we do have our great share of self-actualizing clinicians. Most have a special kind of perceptiveness, an ability to see not only the general, the factual, the abstract, and the categorized, but the fresh, the new, the idiographic as well. They are relatively more spontaneous and expressive, more natural, less self-controlled and inhibited, with less self-criticism. They are open to life in the larger sense. They are less upset by the unknown, the strange, the puzzling, and indeed may enjoy becoming absorbed in it. Their security is less bound to the measurably certain, the knowable, the safe. There is a lack of fear of their inner impulses and more acceptance of the range of emotions expressed by others.

It has been said that nothing humanly important can be learned efficiently, if at all, unless it somehow meets need, desire, curiosity, or fantasy, unless there is some reaching from within, unless learning becomes, as Aristotle said, "second nature." I believe this to be true not only for the child but also for the clinician. For clinicians, this means doing what they themselves consider important. Can they really skillfully convey what they do not believe to be important? This would mean, also, the institution of processes of educating clinicians that would lead to a readiness to alter set allegiances to methods or techniques judged "group applicable" or automatically prescribable according to set reference points such as age, grade, symptom or pattern severity of stuttering, and similar procedures judged "objective." It would lead, perhaps, to an increasing awareness of the simple reality that, especially where stuttering children are concerned, attitudes are more important than facts.

As I have stated recently, most clinicians agree that because stuttering persons vary enormously, therapy succeeds most when the entire range of behaviors, and not just speech, is taken into account. In truth, it is not really possible for therapy to focus exclusively on speech behavior, although some therapies give that appearance. Regardless of therapeutic approach, the stutterer has feelings about what he is experiencing, just as we do, and these feelings are important, sometimes central forces in therapy. We have long recognized that therapeutic success or failure is often attributable to the emotional relationship that exists between client and clinician, rather than to specific speech techniques. The relationship is the key. The goodness of the relationship between a client and his clinician is important, even in therapies that play it down. For example, the fear is sometimes expressed that human engineering approaches to behavioral change must "dehumanize" the clients exposed to them. Although the possibility exists, especially when present goals and procedures are uniformly applied to different individuals, it may also exist in approaches called humanistic, psychodynamic, or personalistic. If a clinician has sufficient need to dehumanize stutterers he may, unfortunately, do so in any therapy structure. So the client–clinician relationship plays a major role, for good or ill.

Stuttering, Clinical Affections, and Interpersonal Growth

Now what about that old bromide of a question, should stutterers treat stutterers? Who would ask this question and why? Some say, "Well, I wouldn't want a schizophrenic person to do schizophrenia therapy." Were I a stutterer, I would recoil at the association. Of course, very few stutterers are schizophrenic. But the implication of such questions is clear—a person with a perceived problem might have difficulty dealing objectively with another person having *apparently* the same problem. But the implication is not universally true, of course. Some recovered schizophrenics are therapeutically assistive to persons judged schizophrenic. Many recovered stutterers are successful with persons who stutter. And some clinicians with stuttering speech are of course successful with persons who stutter.

It is an old observation that an accurate and sensitive awareness of another person's feelings, a deep concern for another person's welfare without efforts to dominate him, and an open, nondefensive authenticity or genuineness will benefit any human interaction. Self-actualizing clinicians are trustworthy and consistent in some deeply important, personal sense. They are able to express attitudes of interest, respect, caring, and liking. They perceive their clients as having the capacity to grow and as capable of charting much of the course of their own recovery. They reveal congruence in what they think, say, and feel. They are in tune with their own feelings and are able to express them spontaneously, but with little motivation to satisfy personal needs that interfere with therapy. They have a genuine and persistent desire to be of help. They are aware of knowledges and procedures pertinent to the task and are able to evaluate and selectively apply them in a mature manner. Finally, they are not imprisoned by a system of fixed beliefs or methods; fixed systems are noncreative foundations for clinical work.

Interpersonal growth in stuttering therapy occurs in different ways: (1) by improving the skills of speech behavior, (2) by satisfying basic needs, (3) by modifying or removing anxiety, fears, or apprehension, (4) by having self-fulfilling or self-actualizing experiences, (5) by emotional release or catharsis, and (6) by self-understanding. Stutterers vary a lot and some will improve most with a domineering clinician, others with more easy-going ones. All therapies will result in improvement, if only by suggestion, if the client has confidence in the clinician. The clinician will often induce this confidence, regardless of the therapeutic model, by showing self-confidence, vitality, sincerity, ability, and interest. It may be brought about, at least for a while, through gimmickry, showmanship, or pure arrogance, but such instances fortunately are rare.

Creative clinicians have points of view; hopefully they are evolving ones that are open to alternatives. They try to tolerate, respect, and become aware of clinical goodness in the views of others, however unintelligible they may seem at the outset; they hold that neither all of truth nor all of goodness is given to any one individual or approach, and each may derive value from his or her particular perspective. Perhaps we need but be faithful to our own situations and opportunities, making the most of them most humanly, without taking it upon ourselves to impress our own views overbearingly upon others of different orientations.

A Concluding Statement

Somewhere in each stutterer there is a fluent speaker who wants to be heard. In each clinician, there are voices from the past that need to be listened to, even as we try to remain alert for future voices that may assist us in our tasks. The creative clinician and the stutterer in the process of moving from creative insecurity toward increased communicative actualization and fuller humanness are each seeking a new kind of wholeness and integrity. Such creative elements transcend theory and technique. And the ultimate purpose of truly creative endeavor is to satisfy our human hunger for a sense of community with others. The dilemmas, the perils in the human condition and in therapy, are real. We are beset by them or we manage them according to the degree with which we understand and communicate with one another. The ultimate purpose of the clinician is simply to use his or her gifts, to be as authentic as one is capable of being, to become a better instrument for helping and being fully with one another. We are intermediaries through which passes all that we have met and by way of which, hopefully, and in the best sense, others are touched. This hunger for identification, for truly evolving as more fully functioning individuals, and the urge to satisfy this hunger is the impulse behind all creative effort—all creative theory, all creative therapy—not only for the stutterer, but for the clinician as well.

THE RELATIONSHIP OF THEORY TO THERAPY IN STUTTERING

MARCEL E. WINGATE

Department of Speech, Washington State University, Pullman, Washington 99163

The first question posed at this Second Emil Froeschels Conference is, "How do the various theories of stuttering facilitate our therapeutic approach?"

I should like to begin by removing the first word of the question. The word "how" implies a positive answer; I think it is more realistic to ask first whether the various theories *do* facilitate a therapeutic approach.

The relationship between stuttering theory and therapy is a matter that has concerned me for a long time. It is a matter that I think is the proper concern of everyone in the field, simply because it profoundly affects not only speech pathologists and persons in related professions but, more importantly, the patients with whom they deal—and their families.

Unfortunately, it seems that many clinicians remain insulated from an appreciation of the relationship between theory and therapy. As a matter of fact, many people in the field have said to me, quite openly and sincerely, that they are more interested in therapy than in theory. This forthright statement seems to reflect the more common distinction that is drawn between matters thought to be practical as compared to what is viewed as being theoretical.

It is possible, of course, to make a distinction between the practical and the theoretical, but that is not where the issue ends, at least not in this particular case. The statement that one is more interested in therapy than in theory reflects a belief that theory is a separate domain, an area of ideational endeavor removed from the actual activity of therapy. It is, furthermore, an attitude that implies that one can make a clear-cut choice between the two. Persons who express this attitude seem to believe that they carry on (or support) therapeutic activity independent of the cumbersome intricacies of theoretical considerations. In some measure they may be right. Unfortunately, however, this attitude loses sight of the fact that at least some part of what is done (and not done) in therapy is very substantially influenced by theory—most often by some particular theory.

Most efforts to deal with stuttering reflect the influence of theory whether or not one recognizes, acknowledges, or accepts this fact. One functions under the

This paper was prepared for The Second Emil Froeschels Conference on the Problem of Stuttering, Pace University, New York, New York, January 31, 1975.

penumbra of some theory, or parts of a theory, whether or not one is "interested" in theory. To maintain otherwise indicates either unawareness or evasion of the extent to which therapeutic undertaking is infused with theoretic effects.

I suspect that many persons who disclaim an interest in theory are really not so naive as to be unaware that therapy approaches reflect theoretical influences. Rather, it has occurred to me that many persons who disclaim an interest in theory really mean to say one or the other of the following: (1) they are distinterested in theoretical positions other than the one they recognize as subtending the therapeutic activity they employ or (2) they are distinterested in attending to facts and arguments that challenge the theoretic base of their practice.

In the final analysis, no one can justifiably disclaim an interest in theory, simply because so much of what is undertaken in therapy is to some extent influenced—in some cases determined—by theoretical matters.

Anyone who is involved in any important way in working with stutterers should clearly recognize the presence of such influence. Moreover, I believe that anyone concerned with the management of stuttering also should be aware of the *ways* in which theory does influence, or determine, what is done in the course of dealing with the patient and whoever else might be involved in the management process. The latter, of course, turns out most often to be parents.

I believe that an adequate answer to the question of the effect of theory on therapeutic approach should proceed from an appreciation of the nature of theories of stuttering.

The so-called theories of stuttering do not merit that designation in any formal or quasiformal sense. When scrutinized closely they are more like myths than theories. Both theory and myth are systems for providing explanation of events, and have in common that they make assertions about the real world that are not obvious, or proven, or perhaps provable in the ultimate sense. Although the line between theory and myth is not always a sharp one, they can be seen to diverge in certain important ways. Myths are designed simply for explanation, not substantive understanding. They are accounts of events that do not seek to yield knowledge but to provide comfort and esthetic satisfaction. Myths account for events through a number of assumptions, many of which have little, if any, credibility and which are often obscured within the overall account or at least not made explicit. In the final analysis, theory and myth differ in the extent to which the assertions contained within them provide for a careful and credible articulation with reality, and in the degree to which they permit and tolerate inconsistency.

It is not necessary to press the contention that extant explanations of stuttering are more like myth than theory. However, it should be clearly recognized that present "theories" of stuttering typically contain considerable inconsistency, assertions of dubious credibility, and assumptions that are not made explicit. Additionally, they seem designed to yield satisfaction more than erudition.

To put the matter more simply, it can be said that the "theories" of stuttering are essentially guesses based on a good deal of conjecture and speculation. Their relationships to data and evidence are not particularly substantial or clear-cut. In fact, most theories consider only a certain portion of the available evidence, many findings are distorted in interpretation, and other pieces of evidence are simply ignored. Each viewpoint has its own set of favored notions and preferred data; each is selective in the observations to which it attends.

It is not necessary or possible to review here the particular limitations of each theory. Rather, we can discuss briefly certain theoretical positions as exemplary of the problems identified above.

We might well begin with the psychoanalytic interpretation of stuttering. Psychoanalytic theory is clearly cast in the framework of myth. Many of its assertions are credible only through committed belief and most of its assumptions are not made explicit. Its tremendous popularity and its remarkable persistence are testimony to the emotional satisfaction and explanatory comfort it affords.

The remarkable latitude and potential for accommodation inherent in psychoanalytic theory are applied to an explanation of stuttering largely through the leverage provided by the fact that speech involves oral activity. The evanescent interplay of dynamic forces permitted in psychoanalytic theory permits the involvement of the other end of the gastric tube as well, and so a variety of interpretative possibilities can be constructed.

The psychoanalytic explanation of stuttering can claim no persuasive support from case history data, research findings, or therapeutic results. In fact, it is a system that ignores much of the reality of stuttering as we can know it now from the extensive accumulation of information about the disorder.

Similar criticism can be made of other kinds of psychodynamic interpretations of stuttering. Such accounts also present stuttering as an expression of some hidden emotional conflict. Sometimes the conflict is presumed to involve speech activity or some abnormal feelings about speaking. In other views such matters are not important. In either case, the actual stuttering is considered to be the overt manifestation of the covert conflict, in either representational or symbolic form. For instance, the stutterer is believed to harbor unfulfilled dependency needs, and seeks sympathy and love or the stuttering is held to be self-punitive acts expressing the need to atone for underlying feelings of guilt. Other "dynamics" could be cited.

The persistence of such explanations of stuttering are due not only to the explanatory comfort they afford but to their remarkable flexibility as well. Whatever the circumstances might be in any particular case of stuttering, the interpretation can be adjusted to fit the observations. For instance, if a stutterer admits to, or is assessed as having, personal problems it is quickly assumed that his stuttering is one aspect of these problems. On the other hand, if a stutterer gives all appearance of otherwise being a normal and well-adjusted individual, his stuttering (i.e., his "symptoms") can be interpreted as his (inappropriate and ineffectual) adjustment to his hidden problems.

There are many possible combinations of personality and behavioral variables that can be invoked to generate explanations of this kind, and so the interpretative possibilities are great. It is this latitude and adjustability that give such explanatory efforts their appeal and longevity. However, such accounts touch reality only at certain limited points. A considerable amount of research has been addressed to the investigation of stuttering as a personality disturbance. The findings of this research leave little reason to persist in the view that stuttering is a form of neurosis or a psychodynamically based disorder.

We might come at this issue more economically by considering the value and significance of certain hypotheses that show up in several different explanations of stuttering. One of these is the "avoidance" hypothesis, which has found expression in several different forms, all of which involve patent overextensions of the original observation (which can be identified as the "reality"). Avoidance had very humble beginnings in accounts of stuttering. It started out as the report made by certain older (i.e., not child) stutterers that they sometimes attempted to avoid certain words because they somehow believed they would stutter on those words. This testimony was often augmented by the claim that if the word were not avoided it would be stuttered.

The claim that one avoids some word because he might stutter on it is a credible claim. It is even credible to claim that one avoids a word because he is *certain* he will stutter on it. However, this does not mean that unless one avoids a particular word he *will* stutter on it. That is, there is no certainty that a wish to avoid, or a "set" to avoid, a word will lead to stuttering on that word. However, this is the assumption that was made, and it represents the intermediate step in the elaboration of "avoidance" from the level of casual report to the status of explanatory hypothesis. The change in significance of "avoidance" was effected through this implicit, and highly questionable, assumption of a cause-and-effect connection between two events.

The next step in the increased stature of "avoidance" is a curious one and undoubtedly one of the best obscured oddities in stuttering theory. The assumed cause-and-effect relationship between avoidance and stuttering was compressed and shifted. Whereas the previous assumption held that stuttering results from a wish (and/or a set) to avoid a particular word the next implicit assumption was that the stuttering of a word *is* the avoidance, which also is now held to be an avoidance of *stuttering* rather than an avoidance of saying some particular word. Thus we have the famous AAHAR "definition" of stuttering, in which it is contended that stuttering is an "anticipatory, apprehensive, hypertonic avoidance reaction" or stuttering is what the stutterer does trying not to stutter.[1] This was later altered, informally, to the assumption that "nonfluency" is the object of the avoidance.

---

[1] This definition, or its equivalent, has been stated in a number of sources. A good statement of the position is presented in Chapter 5 (especially pp. 216–217) in Johnson and Moeller (1956).

The limitations of this concept have been carried into at least two other theoretical positions. Wischner (1950) attempted to translate this hypothesis into a framework supplied by learning theory. It seems clear that the impetus for this attempted translation was a semantic one, i.e., that the learning theory model also contained the word "avoidance." Beyond this, it is clear that Wischner accepted the original assumptions—that stuttering is avoidance—even though he found it necessary to conjecture a somewhat different object of avoidance, namely the "original noxious consequences" presumed to be inherent in parental disapproval of (normal) nonfluency.

Sheehan (1958) found "avoidance" elsewhere in the psychological literature—in the paradigm of the approach-avoidance conflict. Again, the original assumptions regarding the relation between stuttering and avoidance were accepted; and again the object of avoidance was altered to produce a better fit to the model. In Sheehan's presentation the object of avoidance is alternately speech and silence, and the stutterer is presumed to vacillate between the two. However, there is no adequate explanation of how, or why, the stutterer is intermittently, and variably, visited by this presumed conflict.

The essential point being made here in respect to "avoidance" is that, as it appears in theories, it is infused with implicit, and not very credible, assumptions. One can therefore immediately question the value to therapy of this notion and, as well, the rest of any theoretical structure that surrounds it.

Let us now consider briefly the matter of fear, an eminent feature in the field of stuttering that has had a conceptual career similar to that of avoidance. This topic could easily be developed in considerable detail but we do not have the time, and the essential point can be made rather quickly.

Very many (again, older) stutterers will report that they stutter more when they are uneasy, embarrassed, etc. Some of them will speak of fear, but certainly not all of them. Nonetheless, fear has come to be mentioned very frequently in association with stuttering, and regularly in a cause-and-effect relationship. Because it seems so obvious it is a simple connection to make; in fact, most lay people make the connection quite readily. Theory has dwelt heavily on this seemingly obvious connection and has elaborated its claimed significance. Additionally, fear has acquired increase in stature through the semantic aggrandisement occasioned through use of the term "anxiety" as an equivalence.

The germinal notion of fear has probably reached its most highly formulated expression in the version offered by Brutten and Shoemaker (1967) in which stuttering is presented theoretically as "conditioned negative emotion." At this level the notion of the role of fear in stuttering has been elaborated considerably, but it remains essentially the same as in simpler versions.

It is not necessary to develop here an extended criticism of any of the viewpoints that heavily invoke fear or anxiety; it is sufficient for present purposes to point out that all of them, from the simplest to the most involved, neglect in their formulation that stuttering is also reported to occur—and particularly among children —under conditions of *positive* emotion as well. The preoccupation with negative emotion has thus been at least very misdirecting.

Let us now return to the matter of the relation between theory and therapy. I said earlier that theory influences therapy, whether or not one accepts this connection. In one sense this is only partially correct. There are two dimensions of the relation between theory and therapy. In one of them the relationship is only semantic in depth; there are certain therapy methods that exist independently of any theory. Furthermore, as Van Riper (1954) noted some time ago, one does not find as much variety in therapy methods as one should expect in view of the number of different theoretical positions that exist. That is, similar (or identical) therapy methods are used by advocates of differing theoretic viewpoints—the methods are simply discussed or explained in different terms.

The most important feature to note about these "common" methods is that they have been derived empirically, through working with stutterers, and stem largely from a common-sense base.

A few examples should suffice to illustrate these therapy methods. Helping the stutterer to identify the features of his stutter pattern, to modify this pattern, and to practice a new pattern does not need any theoretic base for either planning or implementation. If a stutterer is sensitive about his stuttering, desensitization, in its various forms, is an obvious antidote to attempt. Encouraging a child to talk when he is fluent, and vice versa, are obvious common sense recommendations. Similarly, making efforts to minimize the number of situations that appear to evoke stuttering just seems like a wise thing to do. Also, one does not need a theoretic base in order to encourage a stutterer to stutter more easily. And so on. In fact, most techniques for modifying stuttering have developed originally without the assistance of any particular theory. I mean to include here the "operant" methodology. As I see it, the contribution of this methodology comes essentially through its emphasis on contingency, which, in less formalized terms, is the equivalent of immediacy. But techniques of this kind have been around for a long time too.

It is in the second dimension of the theory-therapy relationship that one finds actual influence of theory on therapy. This influence takes two forms: one is prescriptive, the other is proscriptive.

Prescriptive influences are ones that follow directly from a theory and reflect its explanation of stuttering. A recommendation of psychotherapy, and whatever this might involve procedurally, is an instance of a very comprehensive prescription. Short of this are those therapeutic activities designed to deal with some particular emotional components presumed to be significant in the etiology and maintenance of stuttering, e.g., fear, shame, guilt, and so forth. Having the stutterer deal with avoidance represents an example that is somewhat more circumscribed in focus. Attempting to divest the stutterer of "animistic notions" is another example at a similar level. Any theory-constrained explanation of stuttering that is made to a stutterer also represents a prescriptive influence. Counseling with parents regarding "their part" in a child's stuttering is another such prescription. In my view the latter prescription is one of the more objectionable influences of theory since it so frequently imposes unjustified accusations.

Some of the therapy activities listed above, as well as others that could be mentioned, may be appropriate in certain circumstances, as determined by individualized consideration. However, basic objections to them arise in respect to first, the uniformity with which they are so regularly invoked, and second, because they are a part of some system that is not well articulated with reality.

Proscriptive theoretic influences refer to the repudiation of certain therapeutic techniques because they are believed to be contrary to the theory or because they cannot be accommodated within it. For instance, the use of rhythm is repudiated largely because its effect cannot be explained adequately. Routinely, rhythm is written off as a distraction that, furthermore, most likely will interfere with "productive" (presumably, theory-determined) therapeutic techniques. Suggesting to the stutterer that he slow down his rate of speech is also repudiated regularly. Most theories do not find a place in their rationale to accommodate decrease in rate as a therapy technique. In fact, some positions contend that telling a stutterer to slow his rate might have the negative effect of creating concern about his ability to speak normally. Suggesting to a stutterer that he practice "difficult" words also does not fit in with extant theories; for some it is, in addition, contraindicated since it is considered tantamount to an admission that there are certain words that really *are* difficult for a particular stutterer to say.

In overview, it seems to me that a consideration of the currently popular theories of stuttering reveals little within the theories themselves, or derived from them, that can be claimed to facilitate our therapeutic approach. To the contrary, I think it is reasonable to contend that theories of stuttering have done more harm than good; that they have impaired, rather than facilitated, effective approaches to therapy. Furthermore, I think it is clear that this situation exists because of the nature of existing theories and the character of their appeal.

There is serious need for a theory of stuttering that is grounded on a broad base of reliable data closely tied to reality. Until such a theory is developed I think it will be best if the treatment of stuttering is conducted on empirical and pragmatic grounds, with clear recognition of the kinds of influences present theories generate. Thoughtful pursuit of such practice may lead to discovery of reality-based principles that will contribute significantly to the development of an adequate theory, which may then in turn facilitate therapeutic effort.

I think that a substantial foundation for a sound and productive theory of stuttering already exists. My answer to the second question posed for this conference identifies what I consider to be the major elements of this foundation, and suggests the direction in which the development of theory should proceed.

References

Brutten, E., Shoemaker, D. *The modification of stuttering*. Englewood Cliffs, N. J.: Prentice-Hall, 1967.

Johnson, W., Moeller, D., (Eds.). *Speech handicapped school children* (2nd ed.). New York: Harper & Row, 1956, Chap. 5, pp. 216–217.

Sheehan, J. G. Conflict theory of stuttering. In J. Eisenson (Ed.), *Stuttering: a symposium*. New York: Harper, 1958, pp. 123–166.

Van Riper, C. *Speech correction* (3rd ed.). Englewood Cliffs, N. J.: Prentice-Hall, 1954, p. 410.

Wischner, G. J. Stuttering behavior and learning: a preliminary theoretical formulation. *J. Speech Hearing Dis.*, 1950, **15**, 324–335.

THE IMMEDIATE SOURCE OF STUTTERING: AN INTEGRATION OF EVIDENCE

MARCEL E. WINGATE

Department of Speech, Washington State University, Pullman, Washington 99163

The second question posed for this conference is, "What level of the communicative process (i.e., phonatory, linguistic, or behavioral) appears to be most important in our attempt to explain the nature of the "stuttering block"?

I will dispose of the third alternative at the outset by saying that I am not at all sure what to understand by "behavioral." The term "behavior" has been used with such breadth of implication—that is, from the miniscule to the molar—and yet with such redundancy, that it has lost a good deal of the meaning I once thought it had. I suspect that in most instances of its use in the professional literature there is something of an intent to convey a sense of objectivity. On the other hand, I think there is also a definite intent to imply that whatever activity is referred to by this term is learned activity. The word has had this significance for many years. In recent times it has assumed the equivalence of "modifiable," which actually is simply more of the same.

The word behavior turns up too often and in usage that is redundant. For instance, including the word behavior is unnecessary in such expressions as "verbal behavior," "speech behavior," "stuttering behavior," and even "aggressive behavior." In fact, use of the word is often more than redundant: it also serves to confound matters. It does not help to objectify or specify; rather, it frequently clouds the issue. To the considerable extent that its use implies learning, a presumption is insidiously introduced. To make the point more clearly, in addition to "verbal behavior," etc., why not speak of "peristaltic behavior," "sphincter behavior," "reflexive behavior," and "brain-wave behavior"?

The word "behavioral" is a very broad generic term and in current usage it is much more connotative than denotative. If one wishes to refer objectively to a certain activity that is to be the object of attention or scrutiny, then one should simply specify the activity clearly.

In contrast to the word "behavioral" the terms "linguistic" and "phonatory"

This paper was prepared for The Second Emil Froeschels Conference on the Problem of Stuttering, Pace University, New York, New York, January 31, 1975.

do identify circumscribed domains of activity that can be discussed as content areas.[1]

A good deal of data has been accumulated that suggests that stuttering involves the linguistic level of the communication process. Actually, some of the more fascinating aspects of investigation in stuttering have been undertaken in this domain, and the obtained data are of the sort that have permitted some intriguing, and quite plausible, interpretations.

The initial inquiry into linguistic features in stuttering was made separately by Brown (1937, 1938a,b,c, 1941, 1945; Brown and Moren, 1942; Johnson and Brown, 1939) and Hahn (1942a,b) at about the same time, the early 1940s. Their studies yielded very comparable findings. These data, and the interpretations proposed about them, were recorded in the professional journals. The matter was then essentially abandoned until the time of an active, though relatively brief, revival of interest in linguistic factors, which developed in the 1960s (Bloodstein and Gantwerk, 1967; Conway and Quarrington, 1963; Hannah and Gardner, 1968; Hejna, 1963; Knabe et al., 1966; Lanyon, 1969; Peterson, 1969; Quarrington et al., 1962; Schlesinger et al., 1965; Soderberg, 1962, 1966, 1967, 1969; Taylor, 1966a; Wingate, 1967).

Anyone conversant with this literature will be aware that certain findings have turned up with considerable regularity. Probably the best known of these findings is that stuttering is related to the grammatical class of words: there is apparently more stuttering on "content" words (nouns, verbs, adjectives, adverbs) than on "function" words (articles, prepositions, conjunctions, auxiliaries). It is also pretty well documented that more stuttering occurs on longer words, on less familiar words, and on words occurring toward the beginning of utterances. It is also quite well documented that more stuttering occurs on consonants than on vowels, although some equivocal findings are reported.

The grammatical dimension has received the most attention in efforts to account for linguistic factors in stuttering. It is an interest that has clearly been affected by theoretic bias. The interpretations made by both Brown and Hahn were profoundly influenced by the theory of stuttering most influential in their time and for many subsequent years, namely, the evaluation theory. Both authors proposed that more stuttering occurs on content words because stutterers evaluate such words as more important (than function words) to the meaning of an utterance. Presumably this evaluation of the importance of certain words creates more concern about producing them fluently, which then occasions more stuttering on such words.

The more recent work on linguistic factors in stuttering has included careful

---

[1] It is pertinent to point out, relative to the preceding paragraph, that one could speak of "linguistic behavior" and "phonatory behavior" and that the only contribution of the word behavior is to add surplus meaning.

attention to certain of the other dimensions and has offered worthwhile observations on the relevant data. However, the predominant interest has remained with the grammatical aspect. Also, the preferred interpretation remains focused in the area of word meaning, in such concepts as "information load."

A crucial matter to be emphasized here is that a theoretical "set," extant from the beginning of the investigation in this area, has profoundly influenced the orientation toward the data obtained in these studies. In fact, theoretic bias can be held accountable for the fact that so little attention has been paid to what was actually the most impressive finding revealed in the original series of studies (Brown, 1938b)—which I have not yet mentioned. This finding was that almost all stuttering occurred on the stressed syllable of a word, regardless of the grammatical or structural characteristics of the word. I wish to emphasize the fact that linguistic stress has been ignored for such a long time, because this inattention to a very impressive finding stands as a particularly good example of how theory has distracted attention from a very significant observation and thereby precluded investigation along a promising dimension.

I think the evidence regarding the relationship between linguistic stress and stuttering continues to be the most important bit of information that has yet been found in the research on linguistic factors in stuttering. Brown's original findings regarding stress have been corroborated by subsequent investigation (Hejna, 1972; Wingate, 1972).

Analysis of the major dimensions of linguistic features associated with increased stuttering reveals that there is considerable overlapping among them. Content words clearly tend to be longer than function words; they are also regularly less familiar than function words; they also occur more frequently near the beginning of utterances. This overlap suggests that the seemingly separate dimensions actually reflect a common quality. It might well suggest that the higher incidence of stuttering on certain words is more an expression of the ease with which a word is said. For example, longer and less familiar words are not likely to be produced with as much facility as short and familiar words. Thus, the difference in stuttering on content words, as compared to function words, might be explained as some function of the difficulty level of the speech act rather than in terms of the meaning of the word or a reaction to its communicative value.

In a general sense greater length and unfamiliarity of words may well contribute "load" elements, in the form of complexity of performance, that tend to make content words more difficult to produce. However, many stuttered words are neither particularly long nor very unfamiliar. So, we must look for a better common element to account for the overlap among the linguistic features' relationship to stuttering.

I think this common element is to be found in the dimension of linguistic stress. The finding that stuttering occurs so frequently on a stressed syllable provides a single focus for explaining the other linguistic dimensions of stuttering occurrence. In connected speech it is the content words that regularly contain the stress peaks, whereas function words rarely do. This explanation can account very neatly for the consistently obtained finding that stuttering occurs so much more often on content words. It can also incorporate the findings of more stuttering on longer words and on less familiar words, since length and familarity are essentially aspects of the content-function distinction. In effect, linguistic stress provides a single, efficient explanation for the findings regarding linguistic dimensions of stuttering occurrence.

Assuming that it is correct to conceive of stress in this central role, it is then possible to account for the immediate, or phenomenal, nature of the "stuttering block" at the phonatory level. To put the matter simply, execution of stress prominences in the speech stream is essentially a phonatory function; that is, the expression of linguistic stress is a function of an increased energizing of several actions fundamental to phonation. It should be noted that this explanation clearly reflects a performance (i.e., motor, physiological) difficulty rather than a reactive (i.e., psychological) one.

There is considerable support from other sources for this view that stuttering is best understood as some disturbance in phonatory function. In two articles that appeared in the *Journal of Speech and Hearing Research* a few years ago (Wingate, 1969; 1970) I presented an analysis of the many diverse conditions known to have an ameliorative effect on stuttering. The major conditions considered were singing, speaking to rhythm, choral speaking, shadowing, speaking under masking noise, and speaking under delayed auditory feedback. The analysis of these, and miscellaneous other conditions, led to the deduction that their beneficial effect on stuttering could be explained economically and effectively by a common principle, namely, the induction of some change in the phonatory activity of the stuttering speaker. This explanation has been the object of a number of subsequent investigations that have yielded supportive findings (Adams and Hayden, 1974; Adams and Hutchinson, 1974; Adams and Moore, 1972; Adams et al., 1974; Agnello and Wingate, 1972; Conture, 1974; Conture et al., 1974; Freeman and Ushijima, 1974; Reis, 1974; Wingate, 1972). Reference should also be made to earlier work reported by Chevrie-Muller (1963) and the analysis presented by Wyke (1970).

There is one remaining matter to consider—the consonant-vowel ratio in stuttering occurrence. It has long been accepted that more stuttering occurs "on" consonants than on vowels. Most of the relevant investigation corroborates this commonly reported observation, although some findings are reported as equivocal.

I think the consonant-vowel ratio in stuttering can be shown to represent an artifact based on word structure and the way in which we have typically perceived stuttering. In regard to word structure, most words begin with a consonant, and most stuttering is found to occur in word-initial position. Regarding the standard perception of stuttering, we identify a repeated phone, or a postured ("blocked") phone—mostly consonants—as the stuttering event. However, one may well question whether the difficulty actually lies at this point. In an instance of repetition the consonant is actually being made well—just too often.[2] In the case of a postured consonant, the phone is essentially made; it would be actualized if the speaker simply moved on. In both cases the stutterer is not moving on. It seems evident, then, that the actual difficulty involves the *following* sound, which is almost invariably a vowel (or dipthong). This is tantamount to saying that, actually, stuttering always occurs in the attempted production of a vowel. More correctly, speaking in respect to the data, stuttering always occurs in the attempted production of a *stressed* vowel.

Since vowels are fundamentally phonatory events the foregoing analysis of the consonant-vowel ratio in stuttering permits us also to incorporate these findings in an explanation of stuttering at the phonatory level. In speaking of vowels as fundamentally phonatory events I do not intend to ignore the shaping movements that distinguish one vowel from another. Perhaps these movements also contribute to the occurrence of a stuttering event. However, such movements are present whether or not the vowel is stressed, but stuttering occurs almost exclusively with the stressed version. Once again, linguistic stress, essentially a phonatory event,[3] emerges as the recurring prominent feature in instances of stuttering.

I do not know of anything else in the vast literature on stuttering that approaches the explanatory power of this single dimension. Its potency is not limited to incorporation of the linguistic elements in stuttering; it can also well accommodate other facts about stuttering, such as the effects of fear and other conditions typically explained in psychological terms.

I do not mean to contend that phonation, expressed uniquely in linguistic stress, is the final word in a comprehensive explanation of stuttering, but it does clearly impress me as the most valuable point of departure for future investigation into the ultimate nature of "the stuttering block."

References

Adams, M. R., Hayden, P. Stutterers' and nonstutterers' ability to initiate and terminate phonation during nonspeech activity. *ASHA,* 1974, **16,** 521 (abstr.).

Adams, M. R., Hutchinson, J. The effects of three levels of auditory masking on selected vocal characteristics and the frequency of disfluency of adult stutterers. *J. Speech Hearing Res.,* 1974, **17,** 682–688.

Adams, M., Moore, W. The effects of auditory masking on the anxiety level, frequency of dysfluency and selected vocal characteristics of stutterers. *J. Speech Hearing Res.,* 1972, **15,** 572–578.

---

[2]In case of consonant combination usually the whole combination is repeated, e.g., st..st..stutter.

[3]Of course the neurophysiologic adjustments necessary to this event are implicated.

Adams, M. R., Riemenschneider, S., Metz, D. E., Conture, E. G. Voice onset and articulatory constriction requirements in a speech segment, and their relation to the amount of stuttering adaptation. *ASHA*, 1974, **16**, 521 (abstr.).

Agnello, J. G., Wingate, M. E. Some acoustical and physiological aspects of stuttered speech. *ASHA*, 1972, **14**, 479 (abstr.).

Bloodstein, O., Gantwerk, B. F. Grammatical function in relation to stuttering in young children. *J. Speech Hearing Res.*, 1967, **10**, 736–789.

Brown, S. F. A further study of stuttering in relation to various speech sounds. Q. J. Speech, 1938a. 390–397.

Brown, S. F. Stuttering with relation to word accent and word position. *J. Abnorm Soc. Psychol.*, 390–397.

Brown, S. F. Stuttering with relation to word accent and word position. *J. Abnormal Soc. Psychol.*, 1938b, **33**, 112–120.

Brown, S. F. The theoretical importance of certain factors influencing the incidence of stuttering. *J. Speech Dis.*, 1938c, **3**, 223–230.

Brown, S. F. An analysis of certain data concerning loci of "stutterings" from the viewpoint of general semantics. Second American Congress General Semantics, University of Denver, 1941, 194–199.

Brown, S. F. The loci of stutterings in the speech sequence. *J. Speech Dis.*, 1945, **10**, 181–192.

Brown, S. F., Moren, A. The frequency of stuttering in relation to word length during oral reading. *J. Speech Dis.*, 1942, **7**, 153–159.

Chevrie-Muller, C. A study of laryngeal function in stutterers by the glotto-graphic method. *Proceedings, VII Congres de la Societe de medicine de la voix et de la parole*. Paris, October, 1963.

Conture, E. G. Some effects of noise on the speaking behavior of stutterers. *J. Speech Hearing Res.*, 1974, **17**, 714–723.

Conture, E. G., McCall, G. N., Brewer, D. W. Laryngeal activity during the moment of stuttering; some preliminary observations. *ASHA*, 1974, **16**, 521 (abstr.).

Conway, J. K., Quarrington, B. J. Positional effects in the stuttering of contextually organized verbal material. *J. Abnorm. Soc. Psychol.*, 1963, **67**, 299–303.

Freeman, F. J., Ushijima, T. The stuttering larynx: an EMG, fiber-optic study of laryngeal activity accompanying the moment of stuttering. *ASHA*, 1974, **16**, 521 (abstr.).

Hahn, E. F. A study of the relationship between stuttering occurrence and grammatical factors in oral reading. *J. Speech Dis.*, 1942a, **7**, 329–335.

Hahn, E. F. A study of the relationship between stuttering occurrence and phonetic factors in oral reading. *J. Speech Dis.*, 1942b, **7**, 143–151.

Hannah, E. P., Gardner, J. G. A note on syntactic relationships in nonfluency. *J. Speech Hearing Res.*, 1968, **11**, 835–860.

Hejna, R. F. Stuttering frequency in relation to word frequency usage. *ASHA*, 1963, **5**, 781 (abstr.).

Hejna, R. F. The relationship between accent or stress and stuttering during spontaneous speech. *ASHA*, 1972, **14**, 479 (abstr.).

Johnson, W., Brown, S. F. Stuttering in relation to various speech sounds: a correction. *Q. J. Speech*, 1939, **25**, 20–22.

Knabe, J. M., Nelson, L. A., Williams, F. Some general characteristics of linguistic output: stutterers versus nonstutterers. *J. Speech Hearing Dis.*, 1966, **31**, 172–182.

Lanyon, L. I. Speech: relation of nonfluency to information value. *Scinece*, 1969, **164**, 451–452.

Peterson, H. A. Affective meaning of words as rated by stuttering and nonstuttering readers. *J. Speech Hearing Dis.*, 1969, **12**, 337–343.

Quarrington, B., Conway, J., Siegel, N. An experimental study of some properties of stuttered words. *J. Speech Hearing Res.*, 1962, **5**, 387–394.

Quarrington, B. Stuttering as a function of the information value and sentence position of words. *J. Abnorm. Psychol.*, 1965, **70**, 221–224.

Reis, R. P. The effects of selected vocal characteristics on stuttering frequency and oral reading times of stutterers. *ASHA,* 1974, **16,** 521 (abstr.).

Schlesinger, I. M., Forte, M., Fried, B., Melkman, R. Stuttering, information load and response strength. *J. Speech Hearing Dis.,* 1965, **30,** 32–36.

Soderberg, G. A. Phonetic influences upon stuttering. *J. Speech Hearing Res.,* 1962, **5,** 315–320.

Soderberg, G. A. The relations of stuttering to word length and word frequency. *J. Speech Hearing Res.,* 1966, **9,** 584–589.

Soderberg, G. A. Linguistic factors in stuttering. *J. Speech Hearing Res.,* 1967, **10,** 801–810.

Soderberg, G. A comparison of adaptation trends in the oral reading of stutterers, inferior speakers and superior speakers. *J. Commun. Dis.,* 1969, **2,** 99–108.

Taylor, I. K. The properties of stuttered words. *J. Verb. Learning, Verb. Behav.,* 1966a, **5,** 112–118.

Taylor, I. K. What words are stuttered? *Psychol. Bull.,* 1966b, **65,** 233–242.

Wingate, M. E. Stuttering and word length. *J. Speech Hearing Res.,* 1967, **10,** 146–152.

Wingate, M. E. Sound and pattern in "artificial" fluency. *J. Speech Hearing Res.,* 1969, **12,** 677–686.

Wingate, M. E. Effect on stuttering of changes in audition. *J. Speech Hearing Res.,* 1970, **13,** 861–873.

Wingate, M. E. Concurrence of stuttering instances and stress loci. Presented in Symposium on Linguistic-Motor Determinants of Stuttering, American Speech and Hearing Convention, San Francisco, Calif., November 20, 1972.

Wyke, B. Neurological mechanisms in stammering: an hypothesis. *Br. J. Dis. Commun.,* 1970, **5,** 6–15.

THE RELATIONSHIPS OF THEORY AND CLINICIAN CHARACTERISTICS TO THERAPY FOR STUTTERERS: A DISCUSSION OF THE MURPHY AND WINGATE PAPERS

STANLEY AINSWORTH

University of Georgia, Athens, Georgia 30601

Although my responsibility is to react, to discuss, to comment, this is difficult, since I largely nodded my head as these gentlemen spoke and thought, "yup, that's right." However, I am glad that I have the opportunity to express some of my own thinking in areas related to these papers.

The two speakers have dealt with some basic principles rather than with "how to do" activities. I believe their approach is good for this kind of conference, since I have an abiding faith that more good can come from understanding principles than from learning recipes. Both authors have made creative suggestions and raised some very challenging questions.

The content of their talks has been very diverse. My initial thought was to develop a broader context within which the papers could be viewed for purposes of a proper perspective. I developed two such frameworks but have concluded that they do not add significantly to this discussion. It is interesting to note, however, that both speakers have dealt with relationship phenomena: Wingate with relationships between theory and therapy; Murphy with the relationship between the personal characteristics of the clinician and therapy.

First, let us discuss Dr. Wingate's talk on the explanation of the nature of the stuttering block. My reaction to his title is that phonatory and linguistic aspects can also be considered as behavioral. Wingate is aware of this, as indicated by his reference to the confusions that the term "behavioral" can create rather than make discussion clear and simple.

The diverse conditions that have an ameliorative effect on stuttering to which he referred might well be due to what he has suggested—a change in phonatory activity—but the lack of permanence of the improvement that is generally attained suggests that we have not yet reached a level of critical importance regarding stuttering. Therefore, the alternative suggestions as to why stutterers have difficulty with certain words or certain kinds of words may have as much validity for understanding the problem as the explanation suggested by Dr. Wingate.

This paper was prepared for The Second Emil Froeschels Conference on the Problem of Stuttering, Pace University, New York, New York, January 31, 1975.

The identification of stuttering as possibly a "phonetic transition" defect is of particular personal interest to me since I tried to approach therapy from this standpoint in about 1941. I noted that many stutterers had no difficulty in making the sound, but that the trouble arose in getting from one sound to the next. My method of handling this ended up being very similar to Van Riper's stop-go technique but with a different explanation as to why it was being done. Like many other ideas, it has only marginal success. We probably have a better example of this transition concept in techniques that attempt to help the stutterer move on through the word rather than getting hung up in one place.

Dr. Wingate's other talk on theory offers some very interesting and challenging statements. I quite agree that clinicians function in some kind of framework that could be loosely designated as theory—even if this is only a group of miscellaneous assumptions at a very low level of consciousness. For instance, many therapy practices actually express the assumption that the stutterer "doesn't know how to talk, so I will teach him." Such an assumption, of course, ignores the fact that the stutterer demonstrates that he knows how to talk in a large percentage of his speech and in 100% of the time under certain circumstances or at certain times. Another assumption that some therapies make is that "no stutterer can be cured" or can become a normal speaker. Perhaps stutterers who have continued to have difficulty into adulthood may seldom attain normal speech, but nevertheless some of them do. Also, perhaps three-fourths of all children who are identified as stutterers "spontaneously" stop doing so and other stutterers "cure themselves" at a rate that challenges the success of clinicians.

The idea of theory as a myth is an interesting concept. It should certainly encourage more close examination of theories that we so glibly recite.

In Wingate's statement that most theories consider only a portion of available evidence, I think it should be noted that most of them are based on the assumption that all stutterers stutter for the same reasons. I am aware that it has been equally as difficult to establish "types of stutterers" as to determine "the" cause of stuttering. However, at this stage of our ignorance, we should not discard the possibility of multiple causation.

I would like to emphasize Dr. Wingate's comments about Sheehan's approach-avoidance conflict theory. This theory is an example of how description that seems reasonably accurate moves into the realm of explanation without really explaining anything. The effectiveness of any therapy built around this theory might be due to factors quite unrelated to the "theory."

The fact that therapies do not seem to differ as much as theories was noted by several individuals as early as 1942 immediately following Hahn's publication of *Stuttering: Significant Theories and Therapies*. It is interesting to note, however, that in recent years there has been a greater effort to develop therapies without a corresponding increase in the number and types of theories. It is not surprising that many therapies are empirically derived, because this is our only solution when we really do not know why people stutter.

It is probably true that proscriptive theoretical influences tend to repudiate certain therapeutic techniques because they are believed to be contrary to the theory. However, there is another good reason for repudiating many of the techniques: they do not work on a permanent basis enough of the time.

I agree that there is a serious need for an adequate theory of stuttering, but I would like to present my own bias with regard to this. It seems to me that a single theory might not be appropriate unless it is broadly enough based to include many divergent specifics to account for stuttering in different individuals and at different times in the same individual.

I assume that each of you has already arrived at his own reactions to Dr. Murphy's talk and that what I have to say may further encourage or discourage you in pursuing the directions that are suggested in this discussion. Personally, I always want Dr. Murphy to explore further his general statements that sound so exciting. How do you do the things that he says ought to be done? For those of you who have not done so I am sure you will be interested in reading the booklet put out by the Speech Foundation of America this past year entitled, *Therapy for Stuttering,* which was mailed to all ASHA members. This contained chapters by Dr. Murphy and myself on changing feelings and attitudes and on the nature of therapy and the clinician. I shall not try to repeat material you can find in those chapters. Rather, I would like to take some of Dr. Murphy's remarks and add ideas to them that you may find useful.

How you see the stutterer says something about *you.* Whether you see him as a reactive being (in Dr. Murphy's language) or as someone in the process of becoming is important and is closely related to what you would be comfortable with in therapy. If you prefer certainty, precision, action and reaction, relatively static progression of events, and if you see behavior as a separate act or bits of acts this will lead you into certain kinds of therapeutic procedures. If you view what is going on between you and the client as movement with general overall change, with some ambiguousness as to results or progress at any one moment, you will be inclined to use a different pattern of techniques. Perhaps most of us combine these two extremes in various ways. The challenge is to do so and to use all levels of therapy creatively.

Similarly, if you can view the therapy itself as a flow, rather than as a series of actions and reactions, you begin to get the concept of using the "now" and the "future" effectively. Dr. Murphy points out that faith is future oriented, but I should say that trust and hope are also future oriented. The now, which so many philosophers tell us we should live in, is not a static concept but an expanding-contracting, fluid and dynamic entity. Sometimes now is a particular brief instant in which you must perform in a certain way. At another time, it includes an integration of your past experience, the present events, and the direction that you wish the future to take. Translated into therapy, this lays the groundwork for seeing yourself and the stutterer as persons who are individualized concentrations of various forms of energy. These energies are interacting and relating in a particular fashion to bring about specific change. The depth of this interaction that you can accept and deal with determines the total effectiveness of this relationship. Very briefly, I would like to spell out some tentative understandings of the nature of this therapeutic relationship. I believe you will see its application in stuttering very easily, but it obviously is something that illustrates all kinds of therapeutic relationships.

Murphy, in his chapter of the most recent Speech Foundation of America booklet on stuttering says, "We have long recognized that therapeutic success or failure is often attributable to the emotional relationships that exist between client and clinician rather than specific speech techniques." Many people have puzzled over the nature of this particular relationship.

Fundamentally, the relationship that affects the effectiveness and efficiency of *whatever* procedures you are using is more than rapport, which seems to be a rather vague or passive something. It is my feeling that there is a dynamic flow of energies that influences outcomes. These energies are effective at different levels of complexity and depth.

First, there is a particular kind of *objectivity* that is necessary and that allows certain things to happen. You are all aware of this particular aspect of the relationship, since it is stressed so much in your training and in interpersonal psychology. The essence of it is the setting apart of your own personality so that your emotions, your concepts, and your attitudes do not become embroiled in the miseries, complaints, confusions, aggressions, hostilities, or attitudes of the client. It is a different role from that of a friend or parent, who *is* involved. It need not be a cold separateness, as we shall see, but it is a distinct setting apart of yourself. It allows you to gently reflect to the client the details of his own nature and problems, uncomplicated by your evaluations, your insistences, your subtle pressures so that he can begin to resolve the problems that he has without being overwhelmed by them. This is not necessarily a Rogerian process that I am suggesting here. I believe this is something that happens in any therapeutic relationship where there is reasonable objectivity. This reflecting process may be accompanied by insights and suggestions from you that facilitate the process, but those do not, ideally, consist of your own biases or feelings. When you do this, you are participating in the therapeutic process without adding a distorting emotional involvement. You can learn many skills and certain attitudes necessary in order to do this better; you probably have already learned to do this a great deal of the time, to some degree or another.

This reflection process carries with it other ingredients besides the fact of the reflection itself. By your words, your intonation, your gestures, your facial expression, your postures, and your vocal quality you add something to this that comes from within yourself. What you add is a product of some additional elements in the relationship.

The second major component of the relationship is a particular *kind of under-*

standing, which *functions at different levels.* In other words, this understanding is not a unitary concept but involves some differences, each of which may add particular contributions to the relationship.

One level of this understanding involves an awareness of the psychological mechanisms at work within the client in relation to his problems. You are aware, for instance, of the degree to which the client is using rationalization, sublimation, identification, expressions of inner conflict, and so forth. How you view these particular mechanisms will depend on the system of personality organization you are using or which you believe in, on how you explain behaviors and attitudes by some personality structure. Suggestions that you make will grow out of this structure as well as from your intuitive insights. If you stop at this level of understanding, you will be able to help some individuals to a certain degree. By knowing these you can make more realistic suggestions or even help him become aware of what he is doing. It is more helpful, however, to go on to the deeper levels of understanding.

A second level of this understanding involves the recognition of yourself in the client's problems and person. Basically, nothing that he displays of himself to you is different from what you can find within yourself. All of us have the same tendencies, the potentials for doing or thinking whatever he might have done or thought. You will need some self-analysis to understand this, but his aggressions, his withdrawals, his desire to escape by whatever means, for instance, are extensions of what you can find in yourself. The important thing is that you can now begin to accept him as a person. That is, you can accept him insofar as you can accept yourself *as you are,* totally. When you are able to do this, your own understanding and acceptance flows back to him as you reflect his own nature and problems to him. This, in turn, adds tremendously to your awareness of the psychological mechanisms he is using and what might be done about them. Initially, this may not always change his behaviors, but it does change the quality of the behaviors. Thus, your relationship begins to be something that promotes healing.

A third level of understanding goes even deeper. It is a recognition, a knowing, a seeing, that all the client's maladjustments, struggles, and behaviors that seem so negative are, in themselves, attempts to uplift the self, to know and to express the self more completely, to expand beyond what now is. This idea is not originally mine. I first heard it expressed by O. H. Mowrer in 1956 at a conference on stuttering in Delray Beach. It is difficult to see in this context the blind addiction to drugs or to constantly exposing oneself to maiming and death through fast automobile driving or to other forms of reckless abandon, or, more specifically, the constant efforts of the stutterer to resist anything that might help him. However, these frantic negative expressions are efforts to escape the unbearable frustration, guilt, and shame from repeated failure to find and to nurture his inner identity. Even those stutterers who are apparently successful outwardly have these elements within them. And when we can see those blind, destructive struggles of all human beings in this light of fumbling efforts toward self-realization, we have a depth of understanding that allows us to get across to the client our acceptance of him—not his specific behavior, but of him as an entity. This level of acceptance goes deeper than the level that was mentioned under the recognition of yourself in the client's problems and person. The knowledge that negative and frustrating behavior represents a struggle upward allows us to react to them more rationally and clearly. It is when all of these levels of understanding (awareness of mechanisms, recognition of self in the client, and seeing the nature of negative behaviors) are reflected continuously to the client that he is able to really begin his own healing. You have set the stage for your techniques and methods to become effective.

A third major element in the relationship is *love*. This is a very special kind of love that does not relate specifically to the erotic, emotional types of love that we usually associate with the term. It is not a function of the interaction between two individuals, but it is something deeper. Here again, this is not an original concept but is drawn from many sources. Murphy, for instance, talks about the necessity for hope, faith, love, trust, and courage to accomplish healing. A speech pathologist was invited by graduating seniors to give an address at one university and chose to use this as her primary element in the total rehabilitation process. Anyone who has been privileged to watch a sensitive clinician at work can see elements of it operating effectively.

This love expresses itself on at least two different levels. The first is a strong desire to help. Some writers see this as a deep "caring" for the client in his need for help. The desire to help must be a product of a recognition that you are doing it because the client needs it, not because you need something, for if you do, you are doing the helping compulsively, to feed your own ego. This is self-defeating and does not express the kind of love that is being referred to here. When you do it simply because it needs to be done, that is one level of expression of this kind of love.

Another level can best be called a transcendent love. This springs from your innermost self, from the central identity that is deeper than the brain, the emotions, the personality, I was surprised the other day to read in a newspaper column by Sidney Harris one recognition of this element of self. This is the element that retains your identity even though all cells in your body have been replaced in the past few years. This is the sameness that you recognize as the self even though you "have changed so much." This is the part of you that can stand aside and watch you think, emote, or behave in so many ways. It is the sense of being that expresses through your amazing and intricate mechanism. As you are able to be in touch with yourself, you can release a force that can be called a "transcendent love." This can flow to the person you are helping at the same fundamental level and then neither one of you is alone any longer. This ingredient, plus the levels of understanding already described, provides the total acceptance and support that enable the client to restructure what he has sent to you about himself and which is reflected back. You have enabled him to acquire what he needs in order to heal himself.

Some people express their therapy principally through one or two of these elements or levels. Some of you are very good at objectivity, and this has some healing power in itself. But you may remain too distant. Some of you are very understanding, but the danger here is becoming too involved so that you become a part of the problem. Some of you apparently unconsciously provide a steady flow of transcendent love that affects all you meet. When others are near you, they feel "good." This, in itself, does not provide long lasting solutions but it is a tremendously supporting element through which you can go further with your therapy. Therefore, the ultimate is to use all three elements and all levels consciously and skillfully. When you add this kind of personal relationship to a professional and competent employment of techniques, methods, and systems of therapy, you have a therapy that will be successful.

DISCUSSION I

Chair: R. W. RIEBER

Floor: Dr. Wingate, you illustrated prescriptive and proscriptive techniques. Where you had the positive approach on the prescriptive technique, illustrating several examples of these aspects involved in the proscriptive,. . .

Dr. Wingate: Excuse me, I don't quite follow the question. When I talked about prescriptive and proscriptive influences on therapy that follows from theory, I intended to incorporate in those two subtitles the idea that there are certain techniques for which theories, or a theory, will prescribe what should be done; and that these prescriptions may themselves be questioned as to whether or not they are a meaningful or an effective approach.

On the other hand, there are proscriptive ones, meaning ones that the theory says should not be done, and which, in contrast to the prescriptive ones, may actually be valuable, worthwhile, and usable. The point is that a particular theory will, because of its structure and what is contained within it, say what should be done or sets the guidelines, the limits, the thrust of what should be done and what should not be done and that on both counts it may in effect be impairing the therapeutic attempt or the therapeutic efforts. It may not contribute to it effectively at all. On both the prescriptive and proscriptive levels, one or the other or both lead to a management that is not an effective management approach. Does that answer your question? Aside from that, there may be things, you know, that are usable, which are not included within the theory, which, in many respects, may become a proscriptive target.

Floor: Am I to understand that in support of your theory—or your hypothesis—that stuttering occurs on stressed syllables, rather than on inital consonants . . .

Dr. Wingate: Yes.

Floor: Toward the end, I got the impression that you said it really isn't occurring on the consonants, but on the vowels that follow. Or were you really saying that to support the syllabification . . .

Dr. Wingate: Both. I was saying in respect to both points, the idea being that . . . well, I did say in explanation that the stuttering occurs as a transition defect, and that in my view it can best be described as an impediment in the effort to actualize the vowel that is stressed.

Floor: I'd like to raise a point that may be an impediment in the effort to get out of the consonant, to release the consonant . . .

Dr. Wingate: I don't mean to contrast the consonant with the vowel and say it's not this one, it's *this* one. Obviously, there is a transition between the two. Something goes wrong in the movement or movements, or acts of movement —whatever is involved there—in the coarticulation effects that are involved in moving from consonant to vowel. That aspect of it is something I do not have a final position on because it's a matter that, I think, is deserving of a great deal of investigation. But what I am focusing on is the locus where it seems to happen and what the major contributions of it seem to be. I think the first major effect is that of the effort to move into a position of stress that does involve a vowel, but that doesn't mean to say that I don't consider the consonant significant or important or involved.

Dr. Murphy: May I react to that also because I'm always interested in trying to marry conceptions from various points of view. If I were to think in my terms of what Nick Wingate has been saying; he was talking about having difficulty in moving beyond the block and moving, in that particular case, from a consonant to a vowel, rather than having difficulty primarily with a consonant, the problem is in moving toward—"moving on" is what he said. I had to remind myself that I could conceptualize this not only on a phonatory level, but also on a multidimensional level because the person, I think, reacts to what has happened to him, including a block on a consonant, and he also, I think, has *feelings* about what has happened and what may happen to him. You can bring that right down to the vowel level in terms of his anticipation of what might happen, which you could term a "future orientation." Is it conceivable that there could be hope or hopelessness attached to that apparently merely phonatory level, which really also occurs at a conceptual level? We can talk about these things in the language of *denotation,* but it's not enough for me, because I don't think I behave simply in the language of denotation; I behave also in terms of, both expressively and receptively, in the language of *connotation.* These words and sounds and attempts and movements suggest things to me that I may not be able to verbalize explicitly. Even beyond that, or at least as part of it, it is a language of *evocation;* oftentimes these sounds and especially stressed ones evoke feelings and sensations and experiences in me that are hard to pin down verbally. I sense this as an important part of my attempts to speak.

Dr. Wingate: I've considered that. But I think it's a search for how well this will fit with previous explanations that are comforting. That is, stutterers will and have reported that they have difficulty with certain sounds, and they report that they have difficulty with certain words. I have accepted this. It has been accepted in the profession as what actually happens, that is, that stutterers have difficulty with certain words. We go on to explain why they have difficulty with certain words; for example, because the word has a certain meaning to them, or because the word is prominent in the speech sequence, and so forth. Now, in the stutterer's statement about his difficulty on certain sounds, or difficulty on certain words, he has conveyed to us his perception of where his difficulty is. That is, that the difficulty is with certain words or it's with certain sounds. But stutterers won't tell you, ''I have trouble with stress peaks.'' In other words, the perception is not there. It's something that's an ex post facto kind of drawing together of an observation or an analysis and a previously developed explanation. That's one major point in direct answer to your question—or my effort to make a direct answer to your question.

The other point I'd like to make is one that is relevant and was precipitated by what Dr. Murphy said, and that is that we have over the years had or accepted too glibly and too completely the matter of the stutterer's reported reaction to his stuttering. We have fully accepted the assumption that the stutterer is consistently, persistently, and universally aware of his stutterings. Actually, what one can discover with not too much directed observation and inquiry is that stutterers are not so aware of their instances of stuttering. They're not hanging in there every time with an awareness of every stuttering event. In fact, even when you direct their attention to their stuttering, they may become more aware of only the more prominent stutterings and still remain unaware of some stutterings that you, as a careful observer, can identify. The stutterer will pass right over them. It seems to me that the perceptual aspect of stuttering, from the standpoint of the stutterer himself, is something that's been much overdone, much overvalued, and much overexplained.

Floor: Your explanation of stuttering as something occurring . . . How does that help, for example, to explain the effect of auditory masking?

Dr. Wingate: Well, there are other variables, too, of that same kind. That is, auditory masking isn't the only thing that will produce increased fluency. You can get it with DAF, singing, speaking to rhythm, and so on. I can't explain to you what changes occur in the phonatory function of an individual undergoing masking. There are obvious ones, such as those identified in the Lombard effect, when he talks with more intensity, more loudly. There's more volume, and obviously there's more energizing of the phonatory function when that happens, but the details of the difference in physiologic function at the level of the larynx is something that I have not had any opportunity to investigate myself, or do I know that anyone has. I think the kind of work that Francis Freeman is doing, and that has been done elsewhere, in respect to examining differences in laryngeal function in stutterers and nonstutterers, and when stuttering and when faking stuttering, and so forth, will provide answers to that over the long period. But at the present time, I can only say that there is some gross kind of change, or some change that we can perceive grossly, and that it is my deduction that this is the explanation for the reduction in stuttering. Beyond that, I can't offer a more detailed explanation.

CONCEPT AND THEORY IN STUTTERING: AN INSUFFICIENCY OF EMPIRICISM

RONALD L. WEBSTER

Department of Psychology, Hollins Communications Research Institute,
Hollins College, Roanoke, Virginia 24020

Work on the subject matter of stuttering suffers from a serious handicap—the questionable technical quality of concepts and theories that are broadcast within both the literature and the professional community. Those fundamental principles of scientific procedure that assure the rigor of ties between concepts and observable events have been systematically neglected. The casual acceptance of, and apparently serious adherence to, terms that carry "surplus meaning" (Reichenbach, 1938) is a practice that is not to be commended or should it be continued. Faulty definitions of concepts and a preference for conceptual schemes that have been established largely through subjective judgment and rational analysis have led to a seriously reduced emphasis on the empirical aspects of stuttering.

Flaws in concept and theory have been carried over into stuttering therapies. The conceptual basis for many stuttering therapies is quite unclear. Conflicting therapeutic procedures are frequently employed (Van Riper, 1973; Williams, 1968). Much of the stuttering therapy that is conducted in this country today consists of a bit of dogma about the approach used, a few techniques for altering aspects of intrapsychic processes, a few additional techniques for reducing struggle behaviors in stuttering, perhaps a dollop of behavior modification, and an abiding faith that the unique personal qualities of the clinician will provide the catalyst that will make the whole process work. Results obtained in therapy are reported with vague, generalized descriptions, if they are reported at all (Van Riper, 1970; Ingham and Andrews, 1973). There is no evidence to indicate that therapies derived from theory are any more powerful in producing positive results than those that were derived prior to the age of theory.

The very nature of human behavior seems to seduce theorists into the belief that the study of any human endeavor requires beginning with complex conceptualizations that take into account the unique cognitive and emotional properties of the human organism. When such an approach is taken, overt, observable responses become curiosities or artifacts to be examined when there is time to do so. This general approach has had great popular appeal (witness the past 50 years of theory

This paper was prepared for The Second Annual Emil Froeschels Conference on the Problem of Stuttering, Pace University, New York, New York, January 31, 1975.

in the areas of psychology and stuttering). While one would not deny the importance of cognition and emotion, an emphasis on these factors forsakes fundamental characteristics of parsimony and directness in dealing with physical events that have been demonstrated time and time again to be necessary for progress in science. Thus, it seems to me that the concepts and conceptual schemes that have passed for theory in stuttering have demonstrated little efficacy in generating either scientific progress or reliably effective therapies. The search for theory has supplanted the search for lawful relationships among independent and dependent variables in stuttering (Webster, 1974). A continuing reliance on untested theoretical assumptions has led to uncertainty in therapeutic practice (Wingate, 1971). In my judgment, the rush to theory was premature and was supported by a variety of factors that had little to do with basic goals in science. If we are to understand the serious difficulties that exist with theories of stuttering, it might be well to examine some of the conditions that may have contributed to the present state of affairs, and to consider the elementary requirements for concept and theory in science.

The concern for theory in stuttering as a vigorous, continuing intellectual exercise began in the middle 1920s, about the same time as the founding of the American Academy for Speech Correction. It is worthwhile to consider the role of theory in association with the needs of a young, developing area of professional activity. Perhaps needs for academic maturity and professional identity superseded the requirements for scientific adequacy in theory construction. This hypothesis merits examination.

One important aspect of the use of theory in the 1920s and 1930s was to call attention to the possibility that methods of science could be brought to bear on the problem of stuttering. The introduction and serious pursuit of theory established the form of science and put the stamp of scientific method upon the study of stuttering. There is no doubt that theory stimulated basic research and a variety of different approaches to stuttering therapy. However, the lack of operational specificity of the concepts in theory, and the lack of methodologies for adequately testing the hypotheses derived from theory, retarded progress. Concepts embodied in theories of stuttering were not well defined, relationships among concepts in theories were vaguely specified, and observations were frequently based on interpretations of subjectively evaluated events. It seems clear that the emphasis on theory in stuttering led to the general form of science, but not to the proper substance. Apparently, other forces were at work that drew attention away from the task of improving the quality of concept and theory in stuttering.

In the young discipline concerned with speech disorders, it is likely that the emergence of theory provided an aura of academic respectability. The cruder, empirical manipulations of commercial stuttering schools had fallen into disrepute. Such methods were tainted and were not the proper study of the new science of speech disorders. The organization of opinion and rational discourse under the guise of theory was judged to be more appropriate than the careful examination of empirical matters. Theory soon became the intellectual currency for exchanges within the academic community. Discussions of theory led to interesting conjectures about stuttering, stimulated thinking and writing about stuttering, and gave an enhanced sense of substance to the emerging discipline. Loosely organized schools of thought developed around different theoretical positions. The disciples of various leaders helped to emphasize the relative merits of their respective theoretical positions and the relative weaknesses of other positions. Academic reputations were established on the basis of new and exciting theoretical notions. Generations of students were trained to recognize that theories of stuttering were numbered among the substantive points of concern within the discipline. The emphasis on theory and the diffuseness of theory sustained the use of rational analysis instead of fostering more adequate empirical research methodologies. Criteria by which data were evaluated were informal and were not particularly stringent.

Theory was part of the "zeitgeist" in those disciplines concerned with human behavior during the 1920s through the 1950s. To be without theory was literally to be placed away from the center of the disciplines dealing with human behavior. With theory as the focal point of interest within academia, it became a goal to be obtained. Theories were created for the sake of having a theory. Evidence for this point comes through examination of the methods of theory construction that have been used in the area of stuttering. The main tools have been those of speculation, rational analysis, and subjective evaluation. There have been relatively few attempts to establish the operational validity of constructs embodied in theories of stuttering. In addition, there seems to have been little or no recognition of the need to establish a broad, reliable data base prior to attempting the development of theories. The approach to theory construction was clearly that of theory-before-data. While it is fair to acknowledge the need for speculation as a stimulus to science, it is also fair to note that the freezing of speculation at the level of theory ultimately reduces the mobility and utility of theory.

An additional function of theory was to provide a logical basis for the treatment of stuttering. In the area of treatment, theory provided a structure from which the practitioner could deduce various forms of therapuetic procedures. Theory probably also provided enhanced believability to the practitioner who would base treatment on the supposed scientific properties of theory. The derivation of treatment from theory also extended the promise of science to those who would treat and those who would be treated. Theory gave creative thinkers opportunities to invent their own treatment methods based upon their personal considerations and interpretations of theory. The apparent trend toward eclectic therapies was fostered by a dependence on theory.

Additional biases toward theory propagation and away from basic scientific research may also have resulted from the service orientation that was present within the discipline. It is likely that graduate programs selected more for students who were clinically oriented than research oriented. The emerging theoretical approaches led to an emphasis on client self-report data and the associated qualitative evaluations that provided "data." The "clinical imperative," to do the best one can with the tools available, probably also stimulated what might be regarded as the incorrect use of theory. If one theory did not seem to fit the case at hand, then another could be adapted to the situation. Theory was tested informally, through subjective personal evaluation, and through logical evaluation of apparent consequences in therapy, which resulted from utilization of concepts embodied in theory. The relatively loose usage of theory became associated with a relatively loose definition of the consequences of therapy. The casual approach to theory and evaluation in therapy seemed to generate the feeling within the community that one's professional opinion was the basis by which both data and theory were evaluated. Somewhere along the way, the idea that concepts and theories were to be tested carefully and empirically got lost or misplaced.

What follows is a cursory examination of some theoretical notions that have been applied to stuttering. There is not sufficient space available here to do justice to the relative strengths and weaknesses of these conceptual schemes. I am merely noting that each class of theory has a problem in the relationship of its concepts to empirical events. By calling attention to the possibility of difficulty with these theories, and by then briefly discussing some of the criteria necessary for adequate scientific theories, it is hoped that the reader will be encouraged to examine conceptualizations about stuttering in terms of these guidelines.

During the past 50 years a variety of conceptual schemes have been advanced to account for stuttering. Among them have been the disintegration theories, the psychoanalytically based theories, conditioned-anticipation theories, cybernetic theories, and learning theories (Bloodstein, 1969; Van Riper, 1971). For the most part, these "theories" amount to unsupported or loosely supported conjectures about variables that might be involved in some way with stuttering (Webster, 1974).

The disintegration theories make plausible guesses about possible internal workings of the stutterer. The concepts of disintegration are interesting, but require more of an empirical basis. Psychoanalytic theories have assumed, rather than demonstrated, the validity of intrapsychic processes. Concepts within this class of theory have weak empirical ties and rely largely on processes of intuition and subjective evaluation. Conditioned anticipation theories are also interesting, but are based largely on one limited aspect of stuttering behavior that is reported by clients or is inferred by the observer. This class of theory presents incomplete considerations of other variables in stuttering, frequently dismissing reliable, empirical phenomena with the label of distraction. The cybernetic theories function more as models (Marx, 1963) than theories. That is, the established form of a working system is identified in one area of knowledge and then is applied to guide the establishment of a conceptual analogue in another area. The concepts in the cybernetic theories are based on few observations and rely on inferences about the properties of hypothetical central nervous system structures. Again, this class of theory is plausible, but more work on the empirical aspects of speech control are required in order to improve the scientific status of such theories. The learning theories, particularly early learning theories, were based largely on intervening variables and hypothetical constructs. The empirical bases of constructs in learning theories were not reestablished when attempts were made to apply these concepts to stuttering. Because the learning theories were derived from a laboratory background, it was sometimes felt that to use theory was to use the best available science of the day. Unfortunately, the constructs were far removed from empirical operations that applied to stuttering. Even the well-developed empirical procedures of operant conditioning, which were carefully derived within the laboratory, have been translated into a series of conceptual conjectures in the domain of stuttering.

The current, rather confused and incomplete state of theoretical development within stuttering has probably been unavoidable. There appear to be certain general developmental trends in the push to maturity within the sciences (Conant, 1951). Present conditions seem to represent a necessary step in the development of a subject matter in which methods of science have been newly applied. For example, Marx (1963) has pointed out that concepts introduced in the early stages of scientific development may be loosely specified or may carry surplus meaning. This qualification clearly applies to our existing theories of stuttering. Marx goes on to point out that in order for progress to occur, concepts must be improved by grounding them more firmly in solid empirical observations or by replacing them by other concepts that are more closely tied to data. It would serve us well if, in our consideration of concepts and conceptual schemes that pertain to stuttering, we recognize that the distinctive quality of scientific thought lies in the rigorous specification of explicit relationships between observations and concepts.

William James (Conant, 1951, p. 32) called attention to our use of concepts with these words: "The intellectual life of man consists almost wholly in his substitution of a conceptual order for the perceptual order in which his experience originally comes. . . ." James went on to say that in human experience, concepts and percepts intermingle in important ways. Both elements are necessary in order to develop an understanding of the world around us. Concept without percept amounts to delusion; percept without concept amounts to little more than a fleeting experience—a few images flash before us and are then gone.

There are certain criteria that must be considered in the evaluation of scientific concepts and theories. Some of these essential properties are noted below.

The procedures used in the definition of scientific concepts are particularly important. The preferred definitional method is that of the operational definition (Bridgman, 1927; Stevens, 1939). Concepts are defined by their relationship to empirically specifiable events. Terms are not defined merely by words. A given term is defined by a specific set of procedures and a specific outcome. The meaning of a construct is tied directly to the operations that generate the observable conditions necessary for the inference of that concept. The rigor with which constructs are tied to empirical events is a determinant of the concept's adequacy. In the early stages of scientific development, definitions of constructs may be rather diffuse. However, in order for successful development to occur, ties between concept and operations must be strengthened. The requirement of operational definitions in scientific concepts assures us that we are dealing with palpable events and not mere fictions.

A second critical property of good scientific theory is that of parsimony (Bachrach, 1972). In theory construction, it is generally desirable to employ the smallest number of constructs to account for existing data. Complicated conceptualizations and excessive verbiage are not seen as virtues. The properties of parsimony often stand out with great clarity when we reflect upon the development of the great ideas in science: we live in a sea of air, the planets revolve around the sun, charactierstics that enable the survival of given organisms are fundamental to evolution. The elegant simplicity of these conceptual schemes stands in contradistinction to the complexity and diffuseness of the prescientific speculations that were their immediate predecessors.

An additional desirable property of theory is that of inclusiveness. The theory that encompasses within its structure the widest range of data and still sustains the properties of rigor in conceptual definition and parsimony is the preferred theory. The explanatory properties of theory are often largely a function of their inclusiveness.

Of particular importance in proper scientific theory is the requirement that hypotheses that result from logical manipulations of the theory can be verified. Verification requires the empirical confirmation of predictions derived from the theory. Neither logical consistency nor subjective personal experience would generally be regarded to represent acceptable modes of hypothesis confirmation. The requirement of verification is a requirement for interobserver reliability in detecting and recording phenomena of interest.

Still another necessary property of scientific theory is that of utility. The theory should serve as a useful tool in generating new observations and/or experiments. In stuttering, one might expect that the utility aspect of theory would not only be represented by predictions in research, but also by the efficacy of theory in generating reliably effective therapies.

Finally, for this brief summary, there is one additional property of good theory that we might label "vitality." When a theory displays vitality, the recognition is clear that the conceptual scheme is a working tool that may be continually subjected to modification as new data are presented. The vital theory maintains all the prior conditions stated as being requisite for good theory, even though it may be in a state of flux. In a vital theory, the modifications that result from the feedback of experimentation in observation is a continuing process. Theories lose their vitality if they become hardened structures and begin to impose barriers between themselves and different types of data. The problem at this point is that theory beings to dominate data. Vitality goes out of theory as the dogma quotient increases.

It seems clear to me that when we examine existing theories for operationism, parsimony, inclusiveness, verifiability, utility, and vitality, we fail to find a single theory that meets these requirements. Theories of stuttering show serious methodological deficiencies. The allegiance to theory has presented barriers to progress in our understanding of stuttering. I believe we should recognize the limitations of concepts in theories in stuttering. If there is to be a science of stuttering, then the development of knowledge must be based upon the vigorous, careful search for lawfulness and not upon loosely stated theoretical constructs. I believe we need to move away from a dependency on intervening variables, hypothetical constructs, and hypothetico-deductive processes. The basic thrust of our work should be to establish reliable, functional relationships between objectively specifiable stimulus and response events. Instead of using preliminary observations as elements to generate conceptual frameworks that are then logically manipulated, research should be extended by manipulating variables that are accessible to the experimenter. As a data base is created, we should search for relationships among data that lead inductively to the organization of information and to the derivation of straightforward, testable, empirical hypotheses. There should be a reliance upon improving the description of events, extending quantification of the dimensions observed and/or manipulated, and in establishing reliable relationships between stimulus and response events. There should be a minimum of inference about events that cannot be directly observed.

References

Bachrach, A. J. *Psychological research* (3rd ed.). New York: Random House, 1972.

Bloodstein, O. *A handbook on stuttering*. Chicago: Easter Seal Society, 1969.

Bridgman, P. W. *The logic of modern physics*. New York: Macmillan, 1927.

Conant, J. B. *Science and common sense*. New Haven: Yale University Press, 1951.

Ingham, R. J., Andrews, G. Behavior therapy and stuttering: a review. *J. Speech Hearing Dis.*, 1973, **38**, 405–441.

Marx, M. H. (Ed.). *Theories in contemporary psychology*. New York: Macmillan, 1963.

Reichenbach, H. *Experience and prediction*. Chicago: University of Chicago Press, 1938.

Stevens, S. S. Psychology and the science of science. *Psychol. Bull.*, 1939, **36**, 221–263.

Van Riper, C. Historical approaches. In J. G. Sheehan, *Stuttering research and therapy*. New York: Harper & Row, 1970, pp. 36–57.

Van Riper, C. *The nature of stuttering*. Englewood Cliffs, N. J.: Prentice-Hall, 1971.

Van Riper, C. *The treatment of stuttering*. Englewood Cliffs, N. J.: Prentice-Hall, 1973.

Webster, R. L. A behavioral analysis of stuttering: treatment and theory. In K. S. Calhoun, H. E. Adams, and K. M. Mitchell (Eds.), *Innovative treatment methods in psychopathology*. New York: John Wiley, 1974.

Williams, D. E. Stuttering therapy: an overview. In H. H. Gregory (Ed.), *Learning theory and stuttering therapy*. Evanston, Ill.: Northwestern University Press, 1968.

A FEW OBSERVATIONS ON THE MANIPULATION OF SPEECH RESPONSE CHARACTERISTICS IN STUTTERERS

RONALD L. WEBSTER

Department of Psychology, Hollins Communications Research Institute, Hollins College, Roanoke, Virginia 24020

My response to the second conference question is based on our development of the Precision Fluency Shaping Program, an empirically derived therapy for the treatment of stuttering. Information describing the program was presented in a scientific exhibit at the American Speech and Hearing Association Convention in November 1974. A complete report is in preparation that describes characteristics of the program, results obtained with treatment, and follow-up data.

Our therapy program involves a carefully administered, systematic approach to reconstructing the details of articulation and voicing in stutterers. When we discuss the program with speech clinicians, they generally respond first by asking how this program is any different from what has been done for years. The answer is that our program is substantially more detailed and specific in the responses with which it is concerned, uses procedures that are tailored to the establishment and overlearning of new speech responses, and embodies transfer training, which is a continuing, integral part of the program. The program is standardized, yet flexible enough to be adapted to the treatment of most individual stutterers. The usual amount of time spent by clients in training is on the order of 100 hours.

Our purposes in developing the therapy program have been (1) to provide individuals who stutter with the specific motor skills that generate the reliable use of normal, fluent speech and (2) to provide clinicians with a well-tested, operationally defined therapy for stuttering. We do not propose that we have provided any final answer to the treatment of stuttering. However, we do believe that the program constitutes a very significant beginning in the development of standard treatment methodologies for stuttering.

The term "precision fluency shaping" refers to the technical activities upon which our therapy program is based. Clients' speech responses are reconstructed (or shaped) by carefully defined, small, progressive steps to yield normal, fluent speech that can be readily transferred, again by carefully defined, small, progressive steps, from the clinic into everyday life. As was already noted, the therapy

This paper was prepared for The Second Annual Emil Froeschels Conference on the Problem of Stuttering, Pace University, New York, New York, January 31, 1975.

program was developed on the basis of strictly empirical methodologies. Those procedures that worked were retained; those that did not (even though logic and theory said they should) were discarded.

The program consists of intensive, systematic retraining in *how* the client physically forms the sounds, syllables, words, and sentences of his language. A sequence of well-defined "targets" specifies the "microbehaviors" that are involved in the origination of fluent speech. Clients learn how to attain those targets that are associated with different classes of speech sounds. No supplementary fluency enhancing stimuli, such as delayed auditory feedback, white noise, or masking, are used. Explicit knowledge of speech targets and programmed transfer procedures assure that clients reliably acquire and maintain good speech fluency.

This therapy program is based upon repeated observations that reconstruction of "fine-grained" details of articulatory and voicing responses in stutterers results in the establishment of fluent speech. Basic response elements have been identified that generate fluent speech. These elements have been incorporated in the program as target behaviors that are acquired and overlearned by the client. In brief, the program consists of targets and procedures for reliably instating target use in stutterers.

We use the term *target* to refer to a specific gesture or combination of gestures employed in speech production that are characterized by one or more designated properties of position, force, velocity, or duration. Fluent speech results from attainment of targets specified in the program. Targets are concerned directly with the mechanics of speech production. Targets have been *quantitatively* defined for voice onset characteristics that are to be acquired in this therapy. Targets involving articulatory gestures have been *qualitatively* defined. However, sufficient descriptive information is provided to permit the accurate use of such targets in therapy. Clients are advanced from one segment of the program to the next on the basis of performance criteria specified for each segment. Performance norms have been compiled, which aid the clinician in evaluating each client's progress.

We have determined that the gentle onset of voicing constitutes the single most important target in the program. While there are often substantial differences in articulatory gestures that require correction among different stutterers, the common requirement in establishing fluent speech across many different stutterers has been that of improving the precision of control over voice onsets.

Voice onset characteristics are rather subtle and are difficult to observe. We have found that gross training procedures that rely on clinicians' judgments produce unstable use of this target behavior. In order to work precisely with the reconstruction of voice onsets, we developed a small computer, the Voice Monitor, which is used to measure voice onset characteristics during training in the use of the Gentle Onset target. The Voice Monitor gives a reliable, objective basis for establishing the correct use of a fairly small and rapidly occurring bit of behavior. The Voice Monitor aids our therapy by providing immediate, accurate feedback to the client about the correctness or incorrectness of voice onsets made during practice sessions. After receiving initial instructions on a given program segment, the client can practice with the Voice Monitor while the clinician attends to other duties. The Voice Monitor can be set to evaluate the characteristics of each voice onset that occurs during the flow of speech. The instrument does not become a crutch for the client.

The Gentle Onset target is taught in three stages and is coordinated with newly established articulatory targets during the early portion of therapy. At first, the client learns an exaggerated gentle onset of voicing. Next, a somewhat less exaggerated, moderately gentle voice onset is learned. Finally, the client learns to use a gentle voice onset. As the client moves through the program, the new voicing and articulatory targets are transferred into the speech flow. Explicit, carefully programmed procedures are used to insure the reliable transfer of target behaviors into the speech flow.

We have recently completed the acquisition of extensive follow-up data on 200 stutterers who were treated with the Precision Fluency Shaping Program. As I indicated earlier, these data are now being prepared for publication. Briefly, we have found that approximately 70% of the individuals sustained good quality speech fluency. By this, I mean that they maintained disfluency rates that are at or below 3%. There are additional changes in clients' self-perceptions, increases in social activity, and improved self-confidence that occur as a result of treatment. We have follow-up data on clients who have been out of the program for up to approximately 4 years.

Our work with Precision Fluency Shaping encourages me to believe that our understanding of stuttering is likely to be enhanced if we focus very carefully upon the heretofore neglected details of voice onset and articulatory behaviors in stuttering. I believe we are clearly able to develop more effective therapeutic techniques and, at the same time, to generate an increased understanding of stuttering by looking at the details of speech responses rather than by trying to establish elaborate conceptual notions about stuttering. It would appear as if the physically deviant voicing and articulatory responses constitute the basic disorder in the problem of stuttering. We also have observed that perhaps for approximately one-third of the cases, it will be necessary to examine the details of speech-associated respiratory behavior. We have found that instruction in breath control may be necessary in order to permit some clients to establish the correct use of gentle voice onsets and altered articulatory gestures.

I believe we have tended to observe rather gross response characteristics in stutterers. We talk about disfluencies as if they constitute the basic subject matter of stuttering. I suggest that it may be necessary to improve our techniques of observation so we can more adequately specify the characteristics of articulation and voicing in instances of stuttering. We should measure properties of fluent and disfluent speech within the same individual. I believe we must recognize the need to develop an improved set of procedures for observing details of speech behavior. We must increase our sensitivity to the possibility that extremely small units of response may be absolutely critical in the production of stuttering and in the development of effective therapeutic procedures. If we adhere to careful observation of the details of articulation and voicing, and if we search for variables that control such behaviors, it seems likely that we will be able to identify a constellation of very specific factors that are responsible for the production of stuttered speech. I very much doubt that we will make substantial progress until we shift our focus from concepts to directly observable empirical events.

HOW DO THE VARIOUS THEORIES OF STUTTERING FACILITATE OUR THERAPEUTIC APPROACH?

BRUCE QUARRINGTON

Department of Psychology, York University, Downsview, Ontario, Canada

Considering the current ascendency of learning theories in the treatment of behavior disorders, I believe that the question posed might be rephrased by many as "Are theories of stuttering really necessary?" More specifically, the question might be framed as "What evidence exists that stuttering behaviors differ from other behaviors that have been demonstrated to be under operant control?" To suit those favoring a two-factor theory of learning, the last question could be extended to include control by classical conditioning or desensitization.

In these forms the question at issue is not whether theory plays a guiding role in therapy, but what sort of theory is appropriate in the treatment of stuttering. The latter is an interesting question while the former is a trivial one. Almost certainly theory of some sort, however unsystematic or to whatever extent implicit, guides therapeutic practice. Pure empiricism is a myth in treatment and research. The issue of current interest is whether the guiding theory should be one of the general theories of learning or should be some special theory that distinguishes stuttering behaviors from other behaviors and gives specific therapeutic guidance beyond that issuing from general theories of learning. The answer that I propose to offer is that, at the present time, the treatment of stuttering cannot be approached adequately without resort to special theory. This answer should not be construed to imply that stuttering will never be embraced by general learning theory, but is simply a recognition that the facts of stuttering cannot be accounted for by present learning theories.

Studies of normal speakers have shown that speech disfluencies come under operant control with the attachment of rewarding and aversive contingencies (Hill, 1954; Savoye, 1959; Flanagan et al., 1959; Stassi, 1961; Stevens, 1963; Siegel and Martin, 1965a, b, 1966, 1967, 1968; Brookshire and Martin, 1967; Martin and Siegel, 1969; Siegel et al., 1969). When one turns to stuttering behaviors, however, several studies have failed to demonstrate a reduction in stuttering in the presence of negative contingent stimulation (Frick, 1951; Stevens, 1963; Daly, 1967, 1968; Timmons, 1966). Other studies have shown that when stuttering behaviors are differentiated, some behaviors will increase while others will decrease with negative contingent reinforcement (Martin et al., 1964; Quist, 1966; Webster, 1968; Starkweather, 1970). Such findings suggest that normal disfluencies and stuttering behaviors belong to rather different domains and that stuttering does not map well into operant learning theory.

Two-factor learning theory as applied to stuttering by Brutten and Shoemaker (1967) is in better accord with the facts of stuttering, but it too has certain shortcomings. According to this view stuttering behaviors other than repetitions and prolongations are instrumental adjustive responses and accordingly should increase in the presence of contingent reward. It has been shown, however, that a subclass of such voluntary actions termed struggle behaviors significantly decreases under conditions of contingent reward (Patty and Quarrington, 1974). It also is apparent that involuntary repetitions and prolongations are rather different from other sorts of respondently conditioned behaviors. Nonstuttering behaviors that are part of a conditioned negative affective state tend to be stable or to change slowly when evoked continuously or when elicited in the presence of varying contexts. Compulsive rituals associated with phobic reactions, for example, tend to be unmodified, in the short tun, by recent operation of the ritual or by changes in the situational context. The frequency of repetitions and prolongations in many stutterers can change rapidly under apparently constant stimulus conditions (as in adaptation)[1] or with the addition of a wide variety of distracting stimuli. If these additional stimuli are operating as external inhibitors in the classical conditioning paradigm, then repetitions and prolongations are certainly singular respondent behaviors.

It appears more plausible to account for the inconsistencies in the speech locus of repetitions and prolongations and for the sometimes rapid shifts in their overall frequency in terms of the approach-avoidance conflict model of stuttering developed by Sheehan (1953, 1958). While it might be argued that this view of stuttering is still rooted in yet another general theory of learning, it will be maintained here that its elaborated form as applied to stuttering qualifies it as a special theory. Sheehan (1958) proposed that avoidance drives at several levels of psychological organization may participate in the production of stuttering behaviors. This conceptualization involves a number of assumptions pertaining to ego structure and dynamics and to cognitive functioning, which go far beyond the realm of learning theory as it is understood today.

Special theoretical positions such as this account for much of what is known about stuttering and appear to offer guidance as to what, for the individual stutterer, may constitute the optimal treatment approach. It is not my intention, however, to argue the merits of any particular special theory of stuttering, but to consider some hitherto unreported evidence that indicates the treatment need for special stuttering theory and also suggests the need to extend such views to include a component not usually considered in therapy.

---

[1]From a different viewpoint adaptation phenomenon as evidence of stuttering as learned behavior has been examined critically by Wingate (1966a, b).

Very briefly, I would like to report the results of a series of self-cured or spontaneously remitting stutterers accidentally assembled over the last 20 years. Twenty-seven individuals who claimed to have stuttered as adolescents or into adulthood permitted a lengthy interview, which focused on the events and processes involved in their recovery. Methodologically the study has some shortcomings. A fixed interview schedule was not used. The sample is not believed to be representative of stutterers in general, those adults seeking treatment or even stutterers spontaneously recovering. It is a sample of clearly chronic stutterers who attained fluency rather late in development without benefit of professional assistance of any sort. The study has the redeeming value that the results were almost totally discordant with the expectations of the investigator. For example, it was anticipated that a sizable portion of those claiming recovery from stuttering would prove either not to have been stutterers or would be simulating fluency by interiorization techniques (Douglass and Quarrington, 1952). The nature of their reports and observations of their speech behavior indicated that all had been stutterers and had attained normal fluency.

How had they recovered? In agreement with other studies of spontaneous recovery the process was slow (Wingate, 1964; Shearer and Williams, 1965; Sheehan and Martyn, 1966, 1970), in this sample ranging from 1 to 5 years. Recovery was usually initially associated with one or more significant changes in life situation. As often as not these events could be judged as social gains or social losses. What they appeared to have in common was that they represented challenges with which the individual coped successfully and derived an enhanced sense of self-worth. These changes in life situation were seldom perceived as requiring greater demands for speaking or fluency. Despite the absence of few new incentives to speech improvement, the majority of subjects somehow felt less helpless with regard to their stuttering and began doing something about it. At this point I should mention, and temporarily exclude from consideration, a subgroup of seven subjects who did not experience this change in attitude toward their speech and who appeared to do nothing about it, but nevertheless showed a dissipation of stuttering. Of the remaining group of 20 about half claimed that changes in their self-attitudes were of primary importance and about half attributed their recovery to some new approach to the mechanics of speaking. These judgments appeared to mean relatively little since closer scrutiny revealed that early in the recovery period all this group had adopted new attitudes toward speaking situations, new concepts of themselves as speaking individuals. On the other hand nearly all had also made some specific new attack on the speech process itself. The simplicity of these speech changes was striking. Typically the new speech patterns consisted of one principle such as "speaking slowly" or "talking more clearly" or "speaking in a deeper and firmer voice." Their goal was immediate fluency in a speaking manner that they judged as either natural or at least as a completely acceptable way of speaking. This simple approach tended to be in sharp contrast to a new growing awareness of how and under what circumstances stuttering behaviors were occurring. Typically, subjects clung to a single new principle but became aware of a greater range of applicability. Speaking slowly, for example, might have been employed initially in situations were excitement was usually associated with stuttered speech. Subsequently, the subject became aware of situations where external pressures for rapid interaction were present or of situations where silences had formerly prompted impulsive stuttered utterances.

This greater awareness was usually accompanied by a determination that these situations and their old stuttering behaviors should not occur. Contrary to the investigator's expectations only one subject verbalized a developing unconcern about the occurrence of stuttering in the early stages of recovery.

In this major subgroup of subjects the important features of the recovery process appeared to involve increased feelings of self-worth or capability, reduced feelings of helplessness with regard to stuttering, increased awareness of the circumstances and personal behaviors involved in stuttering, and some extremely simple modifications of speaking behavior that was attended with a higher level of fluency. Fluency was not attained quickly, but typically was established in some situations of considerable personal significance and gradually extended to areas of social functioning of greater and lesser importance.

Perhaps most striking in this group of subjects is the apparent central role of cognitive factors in the recovery process and the lesser roles of incentives and new approaches to speech. Motivation for speech improvement did not issue from new external demands but from within. At first these new speech expectations appeared to derive from a cognitive restructuring of self-concepts. With the recovery process underway cognitive factors continued to be of prime importance. Manipulations of speech tended to remain simple while the occasions of appropriate usage became more clearly defined and extensive. Growing awareness of the circumstances and mechanics of stuttering appeared to be important not in leading to new specific alterations of speech, but rather in cognitively revising or reinterpreting speech situations.

In the total sample approximately 40% reported rather regular major oscillations in the frequency and severity of their stuttering prior to and during the recovery period. When asked the period length, the subjects' estimates ranged from 1 to 3 months. Periodicity in stuttering is a familiar but elusive phenomenon (Quarrington, 1956). Sheehan (1969) has seized upon it as an example of the longer oscillations of stuttering that might be associated with social avoidance drives or ego defensiveness in the approach-avoidance conflict model. These oscillations do appear to covary with feeling state, but the causal relationships are unknown. Against this interpretation of periodicity is the apparent lack of correspondence to known social rhythms. It is possible that this periodicity is a biological rhythm, perhaps attributable to genetic factors. In the total sample 55% of the subjects reported stuttering, or a history of stuttering, in parents, sibs, or children. When this feature was related to reported periodicity a statistically significant association was demonstrated ($\chi^2 = 5.21$, $P < 0.05$), which supports this interpretation.

Turning to the seven subjects who were not their own therapists, but apparently recovered from stuttering without primary cognitive changes or deliberate attempts to modify their speech, it is of interest to note that six of the seven reported both the presence of periodicity and a familial history of stuttering.

Risking the hazard of oversimplification, it might be said that the status of the 27 subjects prior to the onset of recovery could be accounted for by three dimensions. One dimension would be that of social and relational avoidances, the second a dimension of helpless attitudes toward stuttering, while the third dimension might be thought of as a genetic diathesis underlying stuttering having an oscillating and declining course over time.

What follows now is speculation as to the implications of this study for the question under consideration. All the subjects except one asserted that they would have undertaken speech therapy if it had been available or if they had known it was available. It is intriguing to consider how they would have fared had they been involved in various forms of speech therapy at the beginning of the recovery period. In the hands of an operant practitioner, for example, would the process of recovery have been speeded up? On the contrary, it seems entirely possible that the speech-directed focus might, for some of these individuals, obscure the social and relational attitudes of central importance in their stuttering problems. It also seems possible that a variety of therapeutic approaches could have undermined their emerging view of themselves as personally responsible and capable individuals. Of course it can be argued that this matter is a hazard of any therapist-patient relationship and is largely unrelated to the theoretical viewpoint of the therapist. While there may be some substance in this argument, it seems self-evident that theoretical views that are not in accord with the actual problems and needs of clients can only work to undermine their initiatives and enhance their feeling of helplessness.

It may also be asserted that operant approaches to stuttering not only modify specific speech habits but also modify more complex behaviors indirectly. Personally experienced modifications of speech operate as important reinforcements of more complex behaviors that in other terminologies might be designated as self- or social attitudes. These are sometimes called the nonspecific effects of behavioral therapies. I am inclined not only to accept such arguments, but to go further as some have (Russell, 1974) and posit that the therapeutic benefits derived from many behavioral approaches lie primarily in their nonspecific effects. In the case of operant stuttering therapy the fluency gains shown in extra-training situations may, in some cases at least, be principally derived from new self-generated attitudes toward self and specific social situations. Insofar as this is the way in which gains are achieved, this therapeutic approach would seem to be a needlessly blind and hazardous way of conducting therapy.

A final line of speculation pertains to the possible genetically based periodicity component present in some stutterers. Is this a factor beyond influence and not requiring attention or accomodation in therapy? This may not be the case. The nature of the changes occurring periodically are not known. It is possible that individuals experiencing these fluctuations are in quite different psychological states at the various phases of these oscillations. On some occasions they may be more capable of certain sorts of therapeutic undertakings than at other times. If this should be the case, then it is entirely possible that therapy unattuned to the current status of the stutterer could result in the learning of new speech and situational fears and also in the enhancement of intrapersonal conflicts. Fransella (1972) has raised questions about the significance of periodicity of stuttering in therapy and has implied the need to take guidance from the client in considering the pacing of therapy. While there is much to be learned about stuttering periodicity, it appears likely that an adequate theory of stuttering will be required to accomodate a nonlearned component of stuttering.

Throughout this discussion the case has been argued for the need to assess and to select individually optimal therapy guided by a special theory of stuttering. The variety of stuttering behaviors and of stutterers appears to require a diagnostic and treatment approach beyond the resources of general theories of learning. While several special views of stuttering appear to be capable of considerable assessment and treatment sensitivity, it appears evident that we await a more adequate special theory of stuttering and perhaps its convergence with a more powerful general theory of learning.

References

Brookshire, R. H., Martin, R. R. The differential effects of three verbal punishers on the disfluencies of normal speakers. *J. Speech Hearing Res.,* 1967, **10,** 496–505.

Brutten, G. J., Shoemaker, D. J. *The modification of stuttering.* Englewood Cliffs, N. J.: Prentice-Hall, 1967.

Daly, D. A. The effect of punishment (electric shock) of signalled stuttering utterances, and both signalled stuttering expectancies and stuttering utterances on the frequency of stuttering. Ed. D. dissertation, Pennsylvania State University, 1968.

Daly, D. A., Cooper, E. B. Rate of stuttering adaptation under two electro-shock conditions. *Behav. Res. Ther.,* 1967, **5,** 49–54.

Douglass, E., Quarrington, B. Differentiation of interiorized and exteriorized secondary stuttering. *J. Speech Hearing Dis.,* 1952, **17,** 377–385.

Flanagan, B., Goldiamond, I., Azrin, N. Instatement of stuttering in normally fluent individuals through operant procedures. *Science,* 1959, **130,** 979–81.

Frick, J. V. An exploratory study of the effect of punishment (electric shock) upon stuttering behaviour. PH.D. dissertation, State University of Iowa, 1951.

Hill, H. E. An experimental study of disorganization of speech and manual responses in normal subjects. *J. Speech Hearing Dis.,* 1954, **19,** 295–305.

Martin, R. R., Brookshire, R. H., Siegel, G. M. The effect of response-contingent punishment on various behaviours emitted during a "moment of stuttering." Unpublished manuscript, University of Minnesota, 1964.

Martin, R. R., Siegel, G. M. The effects of a neutral stimulus (buzzer) on motor responses and disfluencies in normal speakers. *J. Speech Hearing Res.*, 1969, **12**, 179–184.

Patty, J., Quarrington, B. The effects of reward on types of stuttering. *J. Commun. Dis.*, 1974, **7**, 65–77.

Quarrington, B. Cyclical variation in stuttering frequency and some related forms of variation. *Can. J. Psychol.*, 1956, **10**, 179–84.

Quist, R. The effect of response contingent verbal punishment on stuttering. M. A. thesis, University of Minnesota, 1966.

Russell, E. W. The power of behavior control: a critique of behavior modification methods. *J. Clin. Psychol.*, 1974, **30**, 111–136.

Savoye, A. L. The effect of the Skinner-Estes operant conditioning punishment paradigm upon the production of non-fluencies in normal speakers. M. A. Thesis, University of Pittsburgh, 1959.

Shearer, W. M., Williams, J. D. Self-recovery from stuttering. *J. Speech Hearing Dis.*, 1965, **30**, 288–290.

Sheehan, J. G. Theory and treatment of stuttering as an approach-avoidance conflict. *J. Psychol.*, 1953, **36**, 27–49.

Sheehan, J. G. Conflict theory of stuttering. In J. Eisenson, (Ed.), *Stuttering: a symposium*. New York: Harper & Row, 1958.

Sheehan, J. G. Cyclical variation in stuttering. *J. Abnorm. Psychol.*, 1969, **74**, 452–453.

Sheehan, J. G., Martyn, M. M. Spontaneous recovery from stuttering. *J. Speech Hearing Res.*, 1966, **9**, 121–35.

Sheehan, J. G., Martyn, M. M. Stuttering and its disappearance. *J. Speech Hearing Res.*, 1970, **13**, 279–289.

Siegel, G. M., Lenske, J., Broen, P. Suppression of normal speech disfluencies through response cost. *J. Appl. Behav. Anal.*, 1969, **2**, 265–276.

Siegel, G. M., Martin, R. R. Experimental modification of disfluency in normal speakers. *J. Speech Hearing Res.*, 1965a, **8**, 235–244.

Siegel, G. M., Martin, R. R. Verbal punishment of disfluencies in normal speakers. *J. Speech Hearing Res.*, 1965b, **8**, 245–251.

Siegel, G. M., Martin, R. R. Punishment of disfluencies in normal speakers. *J. Speech Hearing Res.*, 1965, **9**, 208–218.

Siegel, G. M., Martin, R. R. Verbal punishment of disfluencies during spontaneous speech. *Lang. Speech*, 1967, **10**, 244–251.

Siegel, G. M., Martin, R. R. The effects of verbal stimuli on disfluencies during spontaneous speech. *J. Speech Hearing Res.*, 1968, **11**, 358–364.

Starkweather, C. W. The simple, main, and interactive effects of contingent and noncontingent shock of high and low intensities on stuttering repetitions. Ph.D. dissertation, Southern Illinois University, 1970.

Stassi, E. J. Disfluency of normal speakers and reinforcement. *J. Speech Hearing Rest.*, 1961, **4**, 358–61.

Stevens, M. M. The effect of positive and negative reinforcement on specific disfluency responses of normal speaking college males. Ph.D. dissertation, State University of Iowa, 1963.

Timmons, R. J. A study of adaptation and consistency in a response-contingent punishment situation. Ph.D. dissertation, University of Kansas, 1966.

Webster, L. M. A cinematic analysis of the effects of contingent stimulation on stuttering and associated behaviours. Ph.D. dissertation, Southern Illinois University, 1968.

Wingate, M. E. Recovery from stuttering. *J. Speech Hearing Dis.*, 1964, **29**, 312–321.

Wingate, M. E. Stuttering adaptation and learning. I. The relevance of adaptation studies to stuttering as "learned behavior." *J. Speech Hearing Dis.*, 1966a, **31**, 148–156.

Wingate, M. E. Stuttering adaptation and learning. II. The adequacy of learning principles in the interpretation of stuttering. *J. Speech Hearing Dis.*, 1966b, **31**, 211–218.

A PSYCHODYNAMIC APPROACH TO THE THEORY AND THERAPY OF STUTTERING

MURRY A. SNYDER

27 Stuyvesant Street, New York, New York 10003

Probably second to man's anxiety about his own death is his fear of being separated from others. Research studies in sensory deprivation and isolation reveal the trauma that befalls the psyche when it feels alone. Stuttering, a flaw in the flow of communication, threatens the individual with such apartness. He fears ridicule, prejudice, rejection, and at the worst, ostracism. His defense in the face of such real or imagined circumstances is to withdraw further, i.e., to set up psychological barriers between himself and others to protect himself from additional anticipated pain. To attempt to communicate with ease and fluency in the face of such perceived threat and defenses conditioned for many years is a virtual impossibility.

The phenomenon of the 'neurotic paradox' has thus been firmly established. The person who stutters now finds himself retreating in the face of his desire to make verbal contact with others (approach–avoidance). He is wrestling with feelings of fear and anger when he would like to experience intimacy and affection.

Speech pathologists and psychologists are in agreement regarding this conflict. Theories about stuttering coming from both professions really center on trying to help the nonfluent person resolve his state of ambivalence.

At first glance, it must be stated that without a specific theory in mind, it is hard to see how a therapy program can be effective. The therapist must have a blue-print image of what he believes the stuttering phenomenon to be and how he can best proceed in order to help his client grow beyond his need for such speech. If he does not, therapy can only be a trial and error experience with improvement achieved in a hit or miss fashion. There are so many variables at work in the therapeutic process—and the stuttering client presents such a complex problem with many unknowns—that the therapist had best have an orientation that will guide him as he proceeds.

The literature is replete with theories on stuttering, especially in the last 50 years. In the early 1900s stuttering therapy consisted predominantly of phonetic drill, relaxation, and sing-song exercises. The emphasis was to do anything that

*This paper was presented at The Second Emil Froeschels Conference on the Problem of Stuttering, Pace University, New York, New York, January 31, 1975.

would, even if only temporarily, demonstrate to the person who stuttered that stuttering could be abated. Amongst the many early pioneers who tried to bring understanding to the 'tongue tied' condition was Dr. Emil Froeschels. It was his belief that stuttering began in the child's search for words and thoughts, a search that creates syllable and word repetitions, the early stumblings being quite normal and to be expected. However, when frustration and the need to make his wants known evoked tension, the tempo of the normal repetitions would be altered, and gradually prolongations in articulation would appear. When the child would be made aware of these repetitions and prolongations, he would begin to inhibit and struggle against what was happening, with anxiety and distortion of personality ensuing. Dr. Froeschels questioned the prevalent therapies of his time. He doubted that fluency could be achieved by practicing any of the parts of speech (breathing, vocalizing sound, articulating syllables), since the person who stuttered could talk normally at times. To concentrate on the stuttering was unwise, since it was this that caused the stuttering in the first place.

Froeschel's theory on the causes of stuttering contains the first suggestions that stuttering is a conditioned response to early verbal experiences. His recognition that the stuttering is aggravated by the child's attention being brought to it hints strongly at what was later the central issue in Johnson's semantogenic theory of stuttering. His reference to the tendency to inhibit and to avoid as the child would attempt to communicate has become the main theme of Sheehan's approach-avoidance theory.

It is my thinking that stuttering is begun and perpetuated by the above three processes. It begins somewhere in the early falterings, which are normal and which the child would probably outgrow if a conditioned stimulus of a most upsetting nature did not present itself. From the ages of one to five, he is going through a period of monumental changes. From a state of virtual helplessness, he has learned to stand and move around in his environment. He learned to do this amidst applause, approval, and ever present encouragement. Every stumble or fall was greeted with a soothing embrace or encouraging response from the two 'giants' in his environment toward whom he was learning to have good feelings. It pleased him to please them because this brought more touching, more affection. He also was learning to move toward things or bring them to him, which made him feel less helpless and more the master of things around him.

He was also doing something else at this time. He was making sounds that, to the best of his ability, were imitative of sounds 'the giants' were making, and this also brought great attention and those 'good feeling' embraces. He was beginning to become a force in his own life. He began to recognize that feeling of aloneness that he felt when he was first born. Many times it would awaken him in the early months and make him cry, and would go away or lessen when he got approval and affection.

But then something very unsettling would sometimes happen. He would now be about 2 years old and he could do more than just make those sounds. He could say words, and he knew that they meant things. He could even use these words in short phrases or sentences. But, for some reason unbeknownst to him, 'the giants' would not smile. They looked sad, unhappy, and sometimes, angry. They would, at times, turn away, and at other times say to him "What did you say?" or "Say it again, darling, but this time, try it more slowly" or "Repeat it after me." He did not understand. What was he doing that made them look that way? Why were they asking him to repeat his sounds or words? He was doing something wrong. 'The giants' were unhappy. They were less approving. He felt sad, unhappy, lonely. He must learn not to do whatever he was doing any more. He will now be careful about how he says those sounds. He will repeat them if necessary in order to get them right. After all, did not they tell him to do that? Maybe if he pleased them, they would love him again and he would not feel as much alone.

The above describes my conceptualization of the genesis of stuttering. It reveals how it is conditioned, the part parents play inadvertently in its beginning, and the onset of approach-avoidance, which the child has learned he must now do in order to speak. It also includes the emotional factors that the child is grappling with as he learns to talk, namely, his efforts to break away from the isolation and aloneness he feels from time to time. It is a paradox that the very act of learning to communicate, which in no small way helps the child out of his apartness, can be the very experience that, if not handled properly, is responsible for many years of feelings of separation from others.

From theory comes the format for therapy. The person who stutters has associated his stuttering with disapproval from others, with feelings of apartness. This has led to feelings of self-deprecation, much anxiety, especially during the act of speaking, covert anger (which, incidentally, whenever released in therapy erupts in a burst of fluency), and a general distrust of most people, including the therapist.

In so many instances, the client begins his therapy by wanting to talk about his stuttering. He is so often almost obsessively concerned about his dysrhythmic speech. Besides, it seems safer to talk about stuttering than about inner feelings, especially when he has tried to keep them hidden and when he does not trust the person sitting across from him.

The therapist must realize that this distrust stems from years of apprehension regarding the reaction of others toward him, originating with the above described responses from his parents. After all, if his parents could not accept his stuttering, why should he expect that anyone else would?

Most crucial to the therapy is the acceptance by the therapist of the person who stutters. If the client is ever going to let go of any of his defenses, he must recognize that such defenses are not necessary with his therapist. The latter may have to tolerate suspicion, manipulation, and, at times, even verbal abuse. He must realize that he is being tested and if he passes, he may begin to get the trust of his client. If trust between the two is not eventually achieved, then the therapy program will fail. They will not then have a chance (1) to break down the original association in the client's mind between stuttering and parental disapproval (the therapist becomes the parent surrogate), (2) to experience stuttering between them with the growing feeling on the part of the client that no criticism or reprimand for this behavior will be forthcoming, and (3) to allow the person who stutters an environment in which it will seem eventually unnecessary for him to engage in approach-avoidance behavior while talking.

Therapy, in effect, is giving the client a second chance. He experienced feelings of rejection and anger with his parents filling him with much anxiety and suspicion. If he can successfully break down the attitudes that keep him defensive and apart, he will be more at ease with others. He will be able to 'reach out' and 'let in', processes that unfortunately have not been part of his experience. The therapist must be the surrogate person. He may have to represent mother, father, employer, teacher, or any other important person who has been threatening to the ego of the client.

In effect, the therapeutic process is designed to accomplish two things: (1) to strengthen and support the client's self-concept and (2) to reassure the client in his interpersonal relationships. It is felt that progress in these two spheres will lessen the anxiety connected with the approach–avoidance conflict and should allow the client the control necessary to produce speech fluency.

I believe that the stuttering block also can best be explained in behavioral terms. But first, what is the stuttering block? Simply stated, it is a hesitation in the flow of speech generally due to an anticipation or apprehension that the word or syllable cannot be said fluently. Johnson once described this by saying that what a person does in order not to stutter is what stuttering is.

I have already described how I conceive the stuttering to have originated. The normal dysfluencies in a young child's speech would have probably disappeared as his speech patterns developed if it were not for the association of parental disapproval with the initial somewhat faltering efforts at talking. The classical conditioning paradigm explains quite clearly how primary stuttering begins. The onset of approach-avoidance describes the beginnings of secondary stuttering.

Since stuttering entails emotional dynamics that are responsible for its specific speech characteristics, it needs a form of therapy that will get at the emotional patterns. The psychotherapeutic experience allows for an ongoing reconditioning relationship that can alter the emotional fixations serving as the energy force that keeps stuttering going.

There are, in addition, situational stress speech experiences that should be considered in therapy. While underlying emotional dynamics are responsible for the stuttering symptom, it is also true that stuttering, in time, produces anxiety. It is probably a fact that nonfluent speech, because of this negative value placed upon it in our society, tends to perpetuate itself. The person who stutters is in many instances stressed with fears and concern about his stuttering, which probably are greatly responsible for the continuation of this symptom. In other words, in the beginning psychodynamics prompted stuttering to appear, which in turn conditioned the person to stutter more, followed by exacerbated anxiety. Psychotherapy, in individual and group form, gives the client the laboratory experience through which, with minimal or no penalty, he can begin to break down the conditioned fears and inhibitions that keep him locked into nonfluent speech.

DISCUSSION II

Chair: R. W. RIEBER

Summary of Video Segments Presented at the Conference by Dr. R. L. Webster

Male, age 28
Pretreatment
  Percent disfluent words
    Reading = 42
    Conversation = 36
    PSI total score = 27

After intensive 3-week
  treatment program
    Percent disfluent words
      Reading = 0
      Conversation = 0
      PSI total score = 5

Two years after the completion
  of therapy
    Percent disfluent words
      Reading = 0
      Conversation = 0
      PSI total score = 5

Male, age 40
Pretreatment
  Percent disfluent words
    Reading = 45
    Conversation = 80
    PSI total score = 51

After intensive 3-week
  treatment program
    Percent disfluent words
      Reading = 0
      Conversation = 2
      PSI total score = 7

Three and one-half years after
  the completion of therapy
    Percent disfluent words
      Reading = 0
      Conversation = 0
      PSI total score = 5

Male, age 9.5
Pretreatment
  Percent disfluent words
    Reading = 28
    Conversation = 39
    No PSI score

After intensive 3-week
  treatment program
    Percent disfluent words
      Reading = 1
      Conversation = 2
      No PSI score

(Audio only) Three years and
  10 months after the
  completion of therapy
    Percent disfluent words
      Reading = 0
      Conversation = 0
      PSI total score = 1

Female, age 6
Pretreatment
  Percent disfluent words
    Reading = no score
    Conversation = 67

Posttreatment
  Percent disfluent words
    Reading = no score
    Conversation = 5

Male, age 27
Pretreatment
  Percent disfluent words
    Reading = 18
    Conversation = 23
    PSI total score = 34

After intensive 3-week
  treatment program
    Percent disfluent words
      Reading = 0
      Conversation = 2
      PSI total score = 0

Editor's Note: *Dr. Webster presented to the Conference "before and after" videotapes of stutterers. These tapes are described above and are referred to in the discussion that follows.*

Dr. Elliot: I just want to mention some data that I think would be interesting to the group. I went down to Hollins College last summer, and for three weeks took the clinicians' training program. At the end of the first week, I called my college president and said: "I'm learning something and I want to apply it." While I was at Hollins, I ran four stutterers through Webster's program under the supervision of Bob Wilkenson. I did what they taught me to do as a clinician. Those stutterers were fluent, really fluent, at the end of the three weeks. I adapted the program to a weekend format, and ran another six people on weekends only—Saturday and Sunday—in the fall. Those six people became fluent. At this time, of the 12 people who have been run, I cannot get in contact with two of them. The other ten I have followed up on. If you've had the good fortune to talk with them, you'll find that they're rather fluent. Of the ten, all of them have a degree of fluency. One of them is having some really rough days, and I would not consider very successful at this time. The other nine are passably fluent, having good days and bad days. I think all nine of them would say, "Our speech is far superior to what it was."

Dr. Starkweather (Hunter College): I think it's important that when we receive "before and after" tapes and hear descriptions of programs that are successful in producing fluency, it's important to understand what the implications of that kind of evidence are. I think it's important to realize that that kind of success does not imply that there are no other ways to achieve fluency in stutterers. But I want specifically to report on a series of videotapes that I saw, which were produced by Dr. Starbuck at Geneseo College, and to describe the therapy he performs and the effect that it has on his population there. His program is quite different from the one Dr. Webster has described, and he is also achieving remarkable success. The stutterers I've seen have been taped before and after therapy. And there are some long-term follow-ups too. The therapy used is a very straightforward Van Riper technique, and the results are so similar to the results that Dr. Webster is describing, that I asked myself—why are there such similar results from therapies that are very different? The first thing that came to mind was that the therapies are not so very different as they might appear. They're very similar in certain respects. Dr. Webster describes his therapy as systematic, detailed in dealing with specific speech productions, transfer activities, and involving a good deal of overlearning. And I don't think he mentioned that it takes place in a residential setting. All of those terms also describe the therapy that Dr. Starbuck does. He's extremely phonetic, much more phonetic than I really believe is desirable with some clients. Treatment is completed in 6 weeks. I think there are about 6 hours of therapy a day. However, he sees 20 clients at a time, in groups; so that, in terms of efficiency, he's comparable to the program that Dr. Webster has described.

Dr. Webster: I would agree that one should be alert to all sorts of possibilities involving the direct manipulation of stuttered speech, and that there might well be a whole family of techniques that produce good speech fluency. I think perhaps we've been insensitive to the possible efficacy of these procedures and that we've hastened to prejudge them on the basis of casually reported old information.

Floor: One of my observations is if there is any commonality between programs, it is that they all eventually end up allowing the stutterer to simply spend more time with the integrity of the syllable itself. There's something very similar, in fact, identical to what Dr. Wingate mentioned earlier in terms of considering stuttering a phonetic transition. What it comes down to is simply allowing the stutterer to spend more time in transition between sounds. I'd like to ask Dr. Webster a question as to whether he uses voice onsets in relationship to transition. Or in other words, does the voice onset predict how long a transition should be into the vowel or the sound? I wonder if he could be a little more explicit?

Dr. Webster: Well, part of what we're doing with these vowel sounds is stabilizing the posture of the vocal tract during the initiation of voicing *prior* to making a transition to any subsequent sounds. With the consonants, we're trying to stabilize the initial articulatory positions to initiate voicing properly and then have the person go ahead and make the transition to the following sound. It's a little more complicated with unvoiced sounds.

Dr. Elliot: I've used Van Riper's technique for 25 years, and "pull-out" was an integral part of it. I think the question is in part related to the difference in what we're trying to do and how you're trying to do it. There are some elements of similarities, but I think when we consider the exact way we do it—to instruct the stutterer and what he feels is his goal in trying to use or to achieve—then they become very different. For example, in pull-out, you're trying to get the stutterer to, first of all, stop a stuttering experience that he's having and to do something about that stuttering experience that permits him to make the decision as to how the subsequent voicing will go. And so, you may start by having him stutter harder. That's what pull-out means. None of that kind of behavior is used in the Hollins approach, because there is no concept of getting rid of moments of stuttering. You never talk about getting rid of symptoms. You never work on a secondary symptom. You never talk about mastery of the stuttering. You never talk about exaggerating the block. You simply talk about the specific targets that represent the specific things you do when you speak fluently. Therefore, it's an entirely different approach.

Dr. Rieber: I might say I very much like the phrase, "the integrity of the syllable." I think it is the essence of the "enigma of fluency." One might postulate a parallel here that the essence of the mind is dependent on the integrity of the individual. I believe both of these ideas complement one another since in order to properly use syllables in communication, the syllables have to be all of one piece, as it were. One must develop a life style that is equally all of one piece. At least that should be our goal if we live a creative productive life.

Dr. Snyder: May I make a comment? I'd like to address myself to Dr. Webster. First of all, I'm in agreement with Dr. Quarrington in that in your comments concerning theory and therapy, it's conceivable that you do not have a formal construct, a prescribed system of hypothesis put together in the form of a theory with accompanying corollaries. But somewhere implicit there must be theory. As Dr. Quarrington indicates, your approach seems to be an implicit awareness as to what produces fluency, and that is your theory.

Addressing myself specifically to what I have heard and seen, I would like to preface by saying, Dr. Webster, I'm most pleased with what you've done and the successes you've come upon. They've been most dramatic. However, there are a few questions I'd like to ask. We have seen the successes. I would like to know about the percentage or number of people who have succeeded as compared to those who have not succeeded. If Dr. Webster could point out to us why those who have succeeded have done so; and those who haven't, why they haven't, this would give us additional understanding. I have said many times to patients that I don't care how fluency is come unpon—namely: if it's necessary for somebody to stand on his head three times a day, and that will produce fluency, I'm for it. And if the full explanation as to cure is in Dr. Webster's approach, I'm for this. I think that that's the most important thing that a therapist must advocate. He must not be for his own particular method—but for whatever will cure the patient. I'd like to know about the percentages of cure. I'd like to know whether what Dr. Webster is producing is fluency—that is, is it curing stuttering or is it a new way of talking, superimposed upon the stuttering? I'd like to know that. I'd like to know more about whether the cure lasts. I'd like to know if the cure is at the expense of the psyche? By that I mean, is additional anxiety brought to the inner state of emotionality in order to produce this fluency? I would also like to know if the person can speak fluently in all interpersonal situations or only in certain such experiences.

Dr. Rieber: I believe it is an extremely important development that professionals in our field today have renewed faith in their ability to help stutterers. It is a fact that for many years, this faith did not exist. This may simply turn out to be another delusionary system. No one really knows. Time, of course, will tell but you can't hurry history.

Dr. Webster: My approach has been rather atheoretical in the sense of formal theory. I'm not really a member of the hypothesis-testing school of science. I'm a member of the curiosity-testing school.

I approach the problem of stuttering with several assumptions. Number one, there may well be some lawfulness between stutterers and response events in stuttering. After we began to find stimulus variables that manipulated stuttering, variables that were empirically specifiable, empirically manipulatable, it seemed as if the first working assumption was pretty sound. As we began to try to replicate various attempts to manipulate stuttered speech with operant and conditioning procedures, at first I started with all sorts of high hopes about the possibility that we might be dealing with something that was based clearly in learning. As I went on, I decided that maybe I was hoping for too much in the assumption that stuttering was learned behavior. So, I simply have modified the assumption to the point now where I would concur that learning is involved in stuttering at least to the extent to which we can use procedures of learning to change the behavior. I don't know whether learning is specifically involved in the establishment of the disorder. I don't know if stuttering is "learned" behavior or not. I have some biases that suggest maybe it isn't, but those are guesses, and I don't want to dignify them by talking further about them.

A comment about cure: We don't really talk about cure, per se. I'm not sure what the word means. I would say that there exists something that we might call a fluency-dysfluency continuum. This fluency continuum, that when we start with a stutterer, he resides primarily at one region of this continuum, toward the dysfluent side. When we finish with him, hopefully, he has moved closer to the fluency side of the continuum. In the conduct of the program, with approximately four hundred stutterers, we have found that about 95% acquire high levels of fluency which are sustained in a great variety of interpersonal situations, including some fairly stressful ones: speaking before public groups, job interviews, and so on. We have substantial third person corroboration of how these people do outside the clinic as well as speech samples that we have collected ourselves. In the follow-ups conducted after people have been out of the program for some time, we're finding that approximately 70% of our cases are sustaining dysfluency rates that are at or below 3%. Durations of speech blockage, if they occur, tend to be very short, sometimes just barely noticeable, whereas, prior to treatment, they may have lasted for fairly long periods of time—thirty seconds or so.

Of the 30% who are in the "what happened?" category, approximately 15% have sustained fairly substantial improvements over their base line dysfluency measures. The other 15% have drifted back toward where they were prior to treatment. Why are they back there? I don't think we trained some of the people as well as we should, because, for some reason, we make errors in the administration of treatment. I think that there are, indeed, a few instances where stuttering was a social tool used to help persons get along in life. I think there are other cases where the behavior seems to be so disturbed that it is terribly difficult to reconstruct. These cases are few in number, but they exist.

I think that what we're doing is establishing the general form of speech gestures that are frequently used by stutterers when they are fluent. That is, when fluent instances occur with stutterers, I think it is because something happens to change the way articulation and voicing are occurring. I think that what we're doing is teaching people how to purposefully form their speech gestures in the manner that generates fluency. We're teaching them how to turn on their voices and to produce articulation gestures in a way that permits the integrity of the syllable to be maintained.

Now, a few words about the psyche. We have made measurements of psychical changes that take place in our clients. We find that people generally become more outgoing and more confident. They generally show substantial improvements in their self-perceptions as measured by the Perceptions of Stuttering Inventory. We see substantial differences in the way they relate to other people. We will frequently find changes in the social life of individuals. That is, clients become more active socially and some seek more challenging jobs. Note that these changes in testings, attitudes, and self-perceptions occur because fluent speech has been established.

I hasten to point out that all we're trying to do here is simply the approach to the treatment of stuttering. We're trying to make explicit for the stutterer those tools which permit the generation of fluency. As we've moved along with the development of the program, we've gotten better at specifying targets and we've made it easier for the client to learn those targets. We're making good progress, but there is a fair distance along this road still to travel.

Dr. Rieber: I'd like to follow through on our discussion, and I think we will be able to cover all these questions as we progress.

This point leads us to a recent paper written by Roger Ingham of Australia. Dr. Ingham discussed this with me very recently and I think it may be of some interest to summarize this information. Ingham did an experiment in which stutterers during treatment were "bugged." In other words, a device was put on them to monitor them in speaking situations, while they were in therapy. The results indicated that this group of stutterers, who were aware that they were being bugged, showed a significantly high agreement between their report of how much they stuttered and the investigators' report. In the second condition, the stutterers were bugged without their knowing it. Here the investigators found a significant difference between the amount of stuttering reported by the stutterer as opposed to the experimentor. These findings pose several crucial issues. How much does the stutterer's introspective judgment regarding his therapeutic improvement as measured by the frequency and severity of his stuttering can we actually trust? This is obviously a crucial issue because it has implications for the psychotherapeutic treatment of stuttering as well as other psychological problems.

Dr. Wingate: I think that sort of finding, which Dr. Ingham has reported on, is consistent with what I mentioned earlier, that we can't really be too sure, when stutterers tell us that they don't stutter when alone or that they don't stutter under certain circumstances, that they are actually able to produce an observation that would be consistent with that of an independent observer were he there to make assessments of the same events. However, I think that in another way, that doesn't vitiate the improvement that stutterers will report to you in terms of their stuttering being less or their fluency being better. I think that we can accept, even though with some reservation, that they are doing better by their own report, since, in some measure at least, they have been prepared to observe themselves more carefully in circumstances other than the therapy session in order to make a report about the improvement in their fluency.

This is kind of connected in a way, and in a way it's not. But it is something that I had wanted to say prior to the time that Dr. Rieber brought up this point. And that is: it occurred to me that perhaps I should take the initiative to say something about therapy, in that I had it come to me from several sources that generally speaking I am looked upon as someone who is more interested in the theoretical aspects and testing of hypotheses than the matter of therapy itself. In a basic sense this is true, but not in the final sense. I think the eventual objective I've had is to search for those principles which would underlie a significant kind of therapeutic intervention. I do think that the principles that I covered in the second paper are ones that do pull together in an integrated fashion the many divergent sources of reported improvement in stuttering. I think it all shakes out when you look at many, many different ways of approaching stuttering that have had a beneficial effect, that it can shake down to focusing around this essential principle that I've talked about in terms of linguistic stress, that Dr. Onuffak mentioned as "integrity of the syllable," which center in the matter of phonetory control and regulation of phonation. And so, I would go on to say that I have made use of these principles in therapy, although not with extended numbers of individuals because my energies have been spread in other ways too. But in my work with stutterers, I have used these essentially simple and, I consider, basic principles. Not simple in the sense of simplistic, but simple in a unitary sense, and which can be approached in a very straightforward manner. I don't feel it's necessary, nor have I found it necessary, to go through any process of shaping, if you want to call it that—I think shaping is kind of a new word that refers to something that has been done many, many times before; it means simply that you're gradually changing something. I don't think it's necessary to go through that process. I think you can go directly to the core of it. I think that Van Riper's approach, for example, eventually gets to that. It's just that he takes a long way around by working on changing the accessories in stuttering, when you could dispense with that business and get right to the heart of it. So, what I do is explain to people that this is where it is. It's right here. And I'm explaining to them something about vocal fold function, how it operates, and how it is involved in the production of the speech stream. I explain that the essential dimension of phonation is expressed in vowel performance, what goes into making a vowel, and how they are undulated and continued in speech, etc., etc. I give them an essentially rational explanation of it, where some amount of demonstration is necessary; but basically we can cover this in a period of an hour. It's the kind of thing that some of my students who are working with children in schools report to me that kindergarteners can comprehend and can follow. From then on, you get people to talk in a manner in which they are intentionally directed to focus on the matter of phonation. And that's where the control is. That's where the stream of speech is. If you learn to control that, you've got the hang of how you should speak. And it can happen very rapidly. People can improve their speech, in essence, overnight. I currently have three fellows I'm working with. Each is different, has a different pattern of stuttering—had a different pattern of stuttering—and severity level. The one that I find most amusing is a fellow who happens to be a French-Canadian. He speaks English with a French accent, but he has intelligible language. He's a man who has stuttered, as most stutterers have, for most of his life. It wasn't a very marked problem. I suppose in terms of percentage, it was somewhere around 25%, and not heavily involved in terms of what went on during the events of stuttering. He grew up in a small town in French Canada and his mother took him to a doctor. The doctor said the stuttering eventually would go away. But it never did. To make a long story short, it really hasn't interfered too much with his life, but he finds now that being an engineer involves more than sitting at a drawing board: it's going to involve his talking to people and talking a great deal more than he felt he was going to have to. So he thought, well, maybe it was time to do something about the stuttering. Anyway, he came and we got started. The explanation that I gave to him included some kinds of terms that would be meaningful to an engineer. For instance, I'd speak to him of the voice as a carrier tone. For him, that means something that he can grasp very well. The main point that I wish to make about him, as representative of these other people, is that he came back the next time, a week later, and I asked him how he had done. He said; "It's magic! All my life I think it is here. But you tell me it is here. And I no longer stutter." The same has happened with other fellows.

One was a technician in the computer center. Another fellow was a manager for a Grant Company store, the five-and-ten chain. This fellow has operated as a management trainee, in spite of the fact that he had very marked stuttering, round 70 percent, and a very odd sort of pattern: a lot of prolongation. When I presented the explanation and demonstrations he was very impressed. He said, "Fantastic! Absolutely fantastic!" He was soon able to develop excellent control, but when he came back a week later he was talking in the same way he did when I first saw him, marked stuttering and the same kind of pattern. I asked him how he was doing with his speech. "Oh, I'm doing fiiiiine," continuing to talk that way as he answered my questions for a while. I said, "You say you're doing fine, but how are doing right now?" And he answered, "Well, I'm not doing very well now." "Why not?" "Well, God, that's a lot of work. It takes a lot of concentration, a lot of effort." I tell him, "Look, let's shift back into it. You know what to do. Go ahead and do it." So he shifts back and now becomes fluent in talking with me. The reason for mentioning this particular case is that I think stuttering therapy *is* a lot of work. And I think the matter of overcoming stuttering is something that, beyond what we can be given from Mother Nature, the rest of it is work. I think that the reason many stutterers don't improve a great deal is that improving is too much like work. And it isn't that important to them.

I think stuttering therapy can be conceived as a form of skill-training, regardless of what you might think of in terms of the ultimate source of stuttering and the ramifications of it. The improvement of stuttering is achieved through various therapies—other than those claiming improvement through psychotherapy

—which have all had to work intentionally in managing the means and manner of speaking. And the person has got to do that, and he's got to be trained how to do it. That is our major objective, and I think my intention in looking for principles has been to find the simplest and best way of going about that. I think that the matter of phonatory control does shape up as being the focus. But it's the same way, I think, as in teaching someone to play golf or ski; there are certain things that a person can do "naturally," but unless he knows how to do it in the way it ought to be done, he's not going to do it very well. When you learn to play a reasonably good game of golf, one of the first things you need to learn is that the club head has to be brought into the ball at the right time. That's where the point of contact is and where the importance of the golf swing applies. It's not in how far back you take the club, or some of the other motions that one can go through. It's in bringing that club head into the delivery at the ball at the right time. Another thing you need to learn is that you take the divot after you hit the ball, not before. And when you're using a wood, you sweep the ball, but with an iron, you hit into it. Those are things that a person doesn't do naturally, that someone who knows about playing golf can teach them. But these things can be learned intellectually and rationally. As a matter of fact, the man who I had instructing me in golf, when I finally decided I needed lessons, didn't bring out those points particularly clearly, and the improvement in my golf game came after reading Ben Hogan's *Power Golf,* in which he emphasized these matters. I didn't have any instructor there telling me what to do, but I could fit in those particular elements into what I did know from what I had been instructed previously, so I improved. But it was largely an intellectual exercise.

What I'm saying is that this aspect of training in therapy is something that needs to be recognized and that we can combine that with an awareness of what the basic principles are and come up to the heart of the matter, and not bother fiddling around with some of the other stuff that, while it can be included, it needn't be.

Dr. Rieber: There is something that we should really clarify before we go any further. Why must the heart of the problem be in the glottis and not in the pineal gland or in the brain or someplace else?

Dr. Wingate: I don't mean to say the heart is in the glottis. I mean to say that the best evidence we have, as I see it from my analysis of everything that comes to me, is that, in terms of the immediate cause, the proximal cause, where it happens, is at that level. That's where things are going wrong.

Dr. Rieber: I am not really sure that I understand the full meaning of your statement. What convincing evidence is there that indicates that the cause of what is going wrong is at the glottal level. Surely you would agree that the necessary program for the temporal and sequential ordering of syllables is not at the glottal level or any other peripheral level, for that matter. Take, for example, "stuttering like symptoms" in the aphasic. Do you mean to suggest that, in this instance, it is at the glottis where things are going wrong?

Dr. Wingate: I'm saying that as far as where the function breaks down or where the operation breaks down, it is at that point. It involves, of course, more than somehow working those things mechanically. It involves, of course, neurologic function, the activity of the cerebrum. But that's what you're working at—not at something else.

Dr. Rieber: If I understand you correctly, all that you say may be simply accidental, that is, circumstantial evidence. After all, with our present-day technology, the only levels that we can adequately observe are the articulatory and phonectitory levels. This should not force us to conclude that the location or place where things are going wrong need be the glottis.

Dr. Wingate: I don't care if it is an accident.

Dr. Rieber: I'm just posing that as a possibility, because I think your reasoning puts too much stress on the peripheral level and does not give enough importance to how the central level integrates with the phonatory and articulatory processes.

Dr. Wingate: What you're saying is, "Look, this isn't important. Let's go on to the fact that this is relatively unimportant. Let's go on to find out what it is up here."

Dr. Rieber: The point that I am trying to make is that it is too simplistic to give more importance to any one level of the communicative process simply because it is easier for you to technologically observe that level. We can point here, there, or to Washington Square, and say, here's where the action is. I can understand that as perhaps one possible approach to the problem.

Dr. Wingate: Well, that's all I'm talking about.

Dr. Rieber: If that's all it is, a possible therapeutic approach, there is no disagreement. On the other hand, if it is used as an explanation for the cause of stuttering, I think it is basically unacceptable.

Dr. Wingate: Well, all I'm talking about is a therapeutic technique.

Dr. Webster: But it also suggests that if you're going to try to analyze what's happening, this appears to be a good place to search when you consider the effects produced when you manipulate other variables.

Dr. Rieber: I agree.

Dr. Murphy: I'm a little to the left-field side of the main thrust of the discussion. But I think the question and the response point up the basic difference, because one side of us is focusing on the publicly observable phenomenon and making the assumption that that is the most important. And from the viewpoint of technique and improvement, I agree. On the other hand, it may not be the most important thing that's happening in terms of the way that the individual is perceiving what is happening to him. That may be up here or in here. So, it's a very nice example of the source sometimes of our differences.

I think that most of us train our clients or our students or our patients in accordance with what we need to train them to be. In a sense, one could make a good case for saying that we train persons who stutter to come into agreement with what we believe as clinicians. This is O.K. I'm just interested in knowing what

I'm training them to believe, and knowing myself, you might say. It's true that when we do a follow-up study on persons who stutter, we want to keep in mind the fact that we have probably trained them to report to us in certain ways. They're going to tell us what we want to hear, if we've formed any relationship with them at all. There is a certain self-fulfilling prophecy that tends to work if we use any method, and we really believe in it deeply, that, I think—we've said it time and time again—that affects the extent to which we get the kinds of results we believe in.

Now, what that points up has to do with theory; it has to do with process; it has to do with method and clinician and stutterer. To me a theory most simply is a way of looking at things. Now, everyone has a way of looking at things. Let's try to keep as aware as possible about the way we think and look at things. And let's take a look at what our assumptions are and what our tenets, principles, our frames of reference, and ways of operating are, and keep them in conscious awareness as much as possible. And they need not be the same. And they will not be the same because we're different. And our needs for theories and ways of looking at things vary as much as our other needs do—if you'll accept the concept of need—or, at least, our ways of behaving are different.

Over twenty-five years ago, I was exposed to a procedure in treating stutterers emanating out of the work of Samuel Robbins. This was a procedure which had seventeen steps. The first step was simply learning how to breathe properly. And from there, it was a matter of learning how to breathe in a relaxed way. The procedure was highly hierarchized and sequentialized. The procedure then would be to begin to initiate tone in the most relaxed fashion possible; we would start with vowels, and then we'd move on to continuant sounds, L, W, R, W, then on to the supposedly more difficult consonants, then on to syllables, then into words and phrases and sentences, and then reading, and then extemporaneous speech. I worked with a large number of persons using that approach, and I found it very successful. I followed up these individuals, however, and there were twenty, twenty-eight, or twenty-nine of them, two and three years later. Their speech behavior as a group at that time had, to me, regressed to the point where I lost some faith in the efficacy of that particular approach.

At the same time, I recognized that the results that I was having with persons who stuttered had something to do with the way I felt about the method, and I realized that the method I was using I didn't feel completely harmonious with. I felt somewhat uncomfortable using that approach. So I searched for something that I felt more comfortable with, which happened to be something more, if you'll pardon the word, "psychodynamic." Others have declared that they have achieved success with that particular approach. I also recognize, however, that something about that approach had to appeal to them deeply, and they had to feel that they were in tune with whatever the possibilities were, and the system, the methods, and maybe the equipment. They had to feel synchronous with all of that.

Sometimes it is assumed that because of the perspective that I often present at meetings, in terms of the interpersonal relationships, that I don't deal with phonological, semantic, or perceptual processes. That's wrong. I'm still using reinforcement procedures from time to time. A way to put this quite succinctly, I think, would be this: when I come into the presence of an adolescent or an adult who stutters, I'm quite likely at the very outset to say: Try to speak as well as you can, and let's see what you're doing in terms of your vocal apparatus, and try prolonging the sound a little bit. See what happens. How does it feel? Have you tried that before? And slow down the rate of speech. I do all of these things. But I don't want to lose sight of the fact that speech is not simply a dissociated function in the human. The purpose of speech, the reason for speech, the reason for the most fluent speech is that speech is communication. Speech is relationship. The reason for the existence of speech is to be in relationship with other people. It's very difficult for me not to think of the import of the relationship factors when I'm working with an individual, whether I'm talking about how he feels about something, or whether I'm talking about the fact that his vocal attack is a little too harsh.

One of the interesting things that happens in a panel discussion of this sort, or whenever any of us get together and have an opportunity to talk and then talk some more, and really get into details, is that we discover some things that are most surprising. Among persons who act as therapists for stutterers, the fact is that so much that we do has so much overlap among us when all is said and done. We do have more in common than we have in difference. We've probably got to search out what those commonalities are, and not focus certainly on differences, not in any antagonistic way.

Dr. Webster: I'd like to make a response with respect to the comment on Roger Ingham's article pertaining to follow-up. I suppose in a way this also relates to Dr. Wingate's comments about the fellow reporting that he had to work to use the new behavior, which generated fluent speech.

First, with respect to Roger's reports. We found in early, less precise versions of our program, when we were less sure of the targets we were trying to teach, that third-person reports (which would be our equivalent to "bugging") were frequently of the sort reported by Ingham's article. That is, people often did less well in the presence of other people than they did in our presence. We found that third-person reports have improved as we improved the specificity and over-all quality of our training. I would caution against overgeneralizing from a study that uses one particular type of reconstruction procedure to other programs based on different procedures. I think this is an empirical question, and I'm very much in favor of studying it. I don't know how you get by with "bugging" people. I'm not really sure I want to get involved with that.

Dr. Rieber: Apparently one can do it only in Australia.

Dr. Webster: Only in Australia! O.K. As we started our work, we had a few cases early on that were quite remarkable. And we thought, Oh, boy! This is the way to do things. It took almost no training with several of these cases. As time went on, we ran into more and different types of stuttering and we learned that we had to develop better and more reliable procedures for communicating details of fluency targets to people that were better than the ones we started with. As we made our procedure more explicit for the client and improved feedback about the adequacy of the responses being learned, we found that it became easier for clients to sustain fluency. Now, as I said, we still have more to learn about fluency targets, how to communicate them, and how to maintain them. We have found that as we improved these procedures our clients found it easier to acquire and sustain good quality speech fluency. It seems clear to me that explicit knowledge of fluency targets provided the key to the reliable use of fluent speech.

Dr. Rieber: Before you go on, just let me clarify something for my own benefit. When you showed us the tapes, and we saw these specific instances of fluency and stuttering and the improvement, now, how did you choose each sequence that you showed us? How much video tape did you have from the various stages that you used? And how did you choose the specific instances that we saw? What were the criteria you used?

Dr. Webster: To start with, we have made video tapes of all clients who have entered the program, with the exceptions when machines fail during an interview. We have before and after samples of all the cases on video tape.

The selection process involved choosing clients who showed stuttering behavior that was typical of people who have gone through the program. I think the main requirement was that they had to show enough stuttering behavior so somebody looking at a short segment would clearly see we had stutterers starting the program. The only other considerations were mainly technical: was a tape good enough so we could dub it with our crude dubbing facilities? These tapes are representative of what people do in the program.

Dr. Rieber: And they were only in front of the therapist or some interviewer that was associated with the training program—that is, these tapes were only taken in the presence of the person's therapist.

Dr. Webster: Well, the follow-up tapes were made, for the most part, by somebody who had not had any association with those people. And for the follow-up studies on two hundred clients, the telephone calls were sprung on people. For most of those cases, it was by somebody who was with our program, but who had never had any contact with these people. This person joined the program after these clients had gone through treatment. We're aware of possible sources of error, and we try to bias against them as much as we can.

Dr. Wingate: What Dr. Webster had to say about people improving with continued practice and work is, I think, very consistent with the point I attempted to make earlier about stuttering therapy being skill-training, and that with any kind of refined skill—even not so refined a skill—practice does improve the performance. And the person has to understand what he should be doing and how the skill works, and then practice at doing it. One can expect that some people won't catch on as well or as quickly as others, that there are certain refinements that certain individuals will need to be worked through or taken through that other persons learn more quickly or learn better as they move along.

But tied to the matter of looking upon stuttering therapy as skill-training there is, I think, the whole matter of the eventual objective and goal, and how this relates to this business of cure. The profession has a very curious attitude toward the matter of cure. On the one hand, anyone in the profession is very suspect of any kind of method that claims cure. All right. I think that's something we should recognize. The fact that anyone in the profession would be very suspect of any kind of a claim of cure suggests, in my appraisal, that no one really anticipates or expects that there is a cure for stuttering.

On the other hand, they will turn around to anyone presenting a particular method, and will demand: What kind of a cure rate do you have? It's again one of these inconsistencies that I think is shot through a lot of what we find in stuttering. On the one hand, you demand something that you—we—inherently don't expect to find anyway. I think it's something that we recognize in two dimensions. One is something that's very often overlooked: It is that within the field of speech pathology, the only kind of communicative defect or problem permitted within the ranks is that of stuttering. Many of the leaders in the field have been and are stutterers, that is, they are not cured stutterers. The reason they are allowed in and allowed to persist in the field is because we all kind of implicitly understand that cure is beyond them just as it is beyond most, probably all, stutterers unless, again, dear old Mother Nature comes into the picture to help us out at the right time.

If someone has an articulation problem or a voice problem, they're encouraged to get that cleared up before they think about going into the field. But someone who stutters is allowed to come into the field and even encouraged to because we've rationalized in some way or other that because they are a stutterer, they have something to offer that we, who are not stutterers, don't.

Now, I don't mean in any way to be poking fun at people who stutter, who are in the profession. I think there are some very good minds and some very good people in this group and all the ones I know personally, I like very much. I think they've valuable contributions, but the point is that the inherent understanding that we have as a profession is that we're not really serious about this business of cure—not that we wouldn't like to be able to do it. In fact, there is the continual search for something that will be a cure, but we're always skeptical. And the reason we're skeptical is because of the tremendous amount of background we have that leads us to be fairly well persuaded that we're not going to make it.

Dr. Snyder: I'd like to say one or two things and address myself to the comment that Dr. Wingate made, namely, that stuttering therapy or moving toward fluency is hard work. I agree completely. Sometimes in my therapy I really come face to face with this, with clients, in that so many of them are self-effacing, overwhelmed with their feelings of inadequacy and defensiveness in a fluent world. At the same time, they have made an adjustment to their own stuttering, in many instances finding that stuttering has certain advantages. I wonder if we have found that sometimes the client, himself, works against his own therapy and makes our job doubly difficult? I've had patients say to me that the moment of their greatest anxiety is when they're fluent, that they're afraid of fluency. I wonder if this is a problem to all of us in addition to the unknowns that we all have to face.

Dr. Wingate: Speaking of being suspicious, there is another dimension on which I'm particularly suspicious—that, of a stutterer saying that his greatest anxiety is when he becomes fluent. I've heard that, but always from second-hand reports. That is, I've never had a stutterer tell me that. And I wonder to what extent those stutterers who do say it have been programmed to say it. I think such ideas are communicated to them in one way or another by someone who believes it. Anyone who has been involved in a close interpersonal relationship, such as that which develops in what we ordinarily call a psychotherapeutic—or even a lower level of counseling—can be aware of the fact that you can get people to say things that are consistent with what you believe. You can do it even in in-take interviews, as a matter of fact. So that I'm suspicious of the extent to which such claims are a true representation of what the stutterer really means or really feels. It may be that someone might say it on an intermittent, haphazard sort of basis, and not mean what a therapist who thinks that way would like it to mean. I remain very suspicious of that sort of thing.

Dr. Rieber: I'd like to make two comments, the first about Mother Nature. I am very cautious when I approach Mother Nature. I've seen a lot of television lately, especially commercials. Mother Nature is pretty vicious when she wants to be, and rather disinterested in man's personal problems. This can be illustrated by a variation on a theme of Pushkin's dream. Pushkin is alleged to have had the following dream: He finds himself walking down a long corridor. At the end of the corridor sits Mother Nature, with her hand on her chin in a thinking position. Pushkin approaches her and says, "Now that I've got you, I believe I know what you are thinking about. You're trying to figure out how to help all these suffering stutterers who have been so miserable all their lives. But why have you taken so long? Why haven't you done it? These people are suffering. Aren't you going to do anything about it?" Mother Nature looked up at him with a contemptuous sneer and said, "I'm trying to figure out how to develop the life span of the flea. Go solve your own problem. I have more important business to attend to."

I believe that the human organism has been given his higher cerebral capacity of symbolic abstraction for many reasons. Nevertheless, one thing is clear: if man is going to survive, it is not going to be vis-à-vis Mother Nature. That is, if man does prevail, it will be due to what *he* does with his life and his environment.

Dr. Wingate: The matter of Mother Nature participating in stuttering recovery

is, I think, a consideration that has gone through stages, the major stage being that
of repudiation of the whole idea. You know, it wasn't too long ago that people in
our profession would shake their heads quite viciously and mutter some kind of
epithets about pediatricians who told mothers that their children would outgrow
stuttering. It was widely assumed that this doesn't happen, that stuttering got
worse. It wasn't until—I've forgotten what year I published that first study on
recovered stutterers—early 'sixties—that a point was made to reject this assumption. But that study didn't give the first evidence of "getting over" stuttering.
There were other sources in the literature buried back in the 'thirties, which
provided evidence of stuttering disappearing, dissipating as a child grew up. Now,
since the time of my article in the 'sixties, we've had other articles that pointed up
the fact that for some reason stuttering sometimes disappears. It seems to me that
the best explanation so far is that this is due somehow to the workings of Mother
Nature rather than anything else. Again, this is the kind of thing that our orientation to stuttering has clouded. That is, no one wanted to look at the evidence for
recovery because everybody knew that stuttering got worse. As a matter of fact,
stuttering doesn't often get worse.

To take it a little further, if one were to accede to the claims about how the young
child reacts to his stuttering, how he supposedly gets upset about it, and then gets
worse and worse and worse, it seems to me that on a logical basis a child starting to
stutter at the age of three ought to be perfectly mute by the time he's seven. And
that just doesn't happen.

Floor: Could we discuss the nonsevere stutterers? As a matter of fact, some of
the programs are only interested in severe stutterers. Yet, there are many, many
people and many children in the schools who are not severe stutterers, severe to the
observer. As a matter of fact, they may not show very many observable signs of
stuttering, but internally they are stutterers. And they are firmly convinced that
they are stutterers. Do you feel that this is something that should be treated?

Dr. Webster: May I make a response to that in terms of observations we've
made in treating stutterers whom we've never seen stutter? We have found that
these "internalized" stutterers respond well to our program. We go ahead and
teach these clients fluency targets using the same procedures employed with other
overt stutterers. While we do not observe fewer disfluencies (remember we never
saw any to begin with), we find that scores on the perception of stuttering inventory
fall into the normal range. It appears as if once the client learns targets he loses his
fear of stuttering.

Dr. Wingate: A brief comment that I would make and that is: why this
messianic need to cure?

Floor: 'Cause they want it.

Dr. Wingate: Oh, they want it. All right.

Floor: I wonder if you could explain to me the suitable means and what is
therapeutic application? And also, did you gentlemen mention the importance of

a stress syllable? And I wonder if you could carry it over into the therapeutic situation? Do you know what I'm asking?

Dr. Wingate: Yes. I think so. Well, the integrity of the syllable is not an easy sort of thing to identify briefly. The essential point is that each syllable that is spoken has what is identified as a nucleus, and the nucleus centers in most syllables in the vowel sound. Moving on to the matter of the stressed syllable, there are certain differences in the stressed syllable in words, compared to the unstressed or nonstressed, which are reflected in changes that are basically phonatory in nature. One is an increase in the volume or the intensity of the sound produced. The other is the duration of the syllable. And the third is a pitch change. Now, all those are matters that involve some change in the way in which the vocal folds are set into and kept in motion. A syllable is not a static thing, but a ballistic type of movement in which there is a set of motions that overlap with what has gone before and what comes afterward. And to maintain the integrity of the syllable is to maintain it in its production as should be produced in the normal fashion. I guess that's as far as I can take it in a descriptive sense at the moment.

Now, how to introduce that into a therapy program? The way in which I introduce it is in terms of explaining to the person, in hopefully simpler terms than this, what's involved in producing a stressed as compared to an unstressed syllable and how the flow of movement should go in the correct or the reasonably correct normal way of moving through a word. It isn't a very hard thing to communicate. You can do it by example, and you can do it by, in essence, choral speaking; by instructing the person in terms of feedback from the vocal folds, the area of the vocal folds. I do make use of having the person hold his throat when he talks so that there is an increase in the matter of direct and additional feedback; thereby his awareness of vibration is increased. And then gradually you can take that away, so that he just gets it directly form the source. Pulling all those things together is the way in which I make use of it therapeutically.

Dr. Rieber: I would like to comment on the importance of the "integrity of the syllable" in fluent communication. I believe that the basic element that holds the word and consequently the sentence structure fluently together is the integrity of the syllable. When fluency fails or falls to pieces, as one might say, this must have something directly to do with (1) a basic timing variable, (2) a basic sequential ordering variable, and (3) a basic cognitive and emotional attention process that facilitates the interpersonal speech act.

Dr. Snyder: I'd like to say something concerning this, if I may. Dr. Wingate said something about golf; I'd like to say something about baseball. I don't know how much you people are learning about stuttering; maybe you will learn a little bit more about sports. I'm thinking when Willie Mays came up to the New York Giants back in 1951—that's going back a couple of years—and right in the very beginning, Willie was having a great deal of difficulty. He had all the phenomenal attributes a star ball player should have. But he wasn't performing well. He went 0 for 20 and Leo Durocher, the manager, said to him, "Willie, just don't worry about anything. You know what you have to do; just get in there and swing." And then, the next time he got up, the twenty-first time, he hit a home run, and that was the beginning of Willie Mays.

To me, the meaning of this is that Willie could have been ruined, I think, if anybody started tampering with his total gestalt as a baseball hitter. To start emphasizing the swing or how he stood at bat was beyond Willie's understanding. Willie was a "natural." I think by and large this is true for all of us. We are all natural in our talking. It's part of the total gestalt of thinking, breathing, and vocalizing. And I'm a little concerned frankly—maybe I don't understand it, this "integrity of the syllable." It sounds somewhat like breaking the whole thing down into its separate components, which I think can be a little bit more than the speaker can juggle. To aim toward fluency is to put this total gestalt of talking together, and this must be emphasized, I think, in therapy.

Dr. Rieber: I think that was the point. It's not that one should break things down into its component parts; on the contrary, the emphasis is on what keeps the whole process in equilibrium without falling apart. It seems to me that you've got to have something to hold it together, and I personally can't imagine any kind of fluent human communication that will hold together without the "integrity of the syllable" (i.e., proper timing, sequential ordering, and attention).

Dr. Snyder: I understand, but I'm talking about the emphasis of it in therapy. Bringing this to the client's awareness can throw him off from the total gestalt necessary in order to speak fluently.

Dr. Rieber: It depends on the way you you do it.

Floor: I have two questions. Is there any point, ever, Dr. Webster, where the pupil or the person in therapy works only with a machine? That's one question. Second question: Do you ever discuss or work directly on secondary characteristics?

Dr. Webster: There are frequent instances during the program where people are talking to a machine and the clinician is not present. This happens only after we've been assured that the client understands the target to be practiced and has been able to demonstrate it properly.

We really almost never do anything with secondary characteristics. They fall out as the client reaches the early stages of the program. It's rarely that they reduce and direct attention. They just drop out.

Dr. Rieber: Another question?

Floor: Several speakers have mentioned differences among stutterers. What are these differences and how does one take them into account in treatment?

Dr. Wingate: The matter of individual differences among stutterers is somewhat different from saying "different stutterers" or "different stutterings" or "different sources of stuttering." We all have individual differences. I think that's another thing that's been lost sight of when we talk about individual differences among stutterers. The implication usually is that the individual differences indicate that the stuttering comes from different sources. Actually the stuttering may have very little relationship to individual differences.

The matter of different sources of stuttering or different causes of stuttering is something that's mentioned from time to time, and it's always an intriguing potential possibility, but there are two major considerations, I think, that bear on the matter. One is that you always get down to the fact that, when you look at stutterers, there is something common to them all and that's the stuttering, and it is fundamentally the same. The second thing is that if one were to try to go about separating different kinds of stutterers, what dimensions would you begin to use to make a separation? I think all efforts so far that might have been tried along those lines have been stymied by that very serious, very insurmountable, obstacle. What are the dimensions on which you would make a discrimination as to which one should be this group, which this group, and so on? In other words, the bases for discriminating differences are more conjectural than realistic.

Dr. Quarrington: I think that there is some evidence that there are some differences that have been demonstrated that indicate that stutterers do respond differently to the same sorts of treatments. For example, in the group that I was talking about today, the spontaneously recovering group, there were very few who claimed to have a predominantly nonvocal form of block, that typically their struggles were vocal in character. I think they were peculiar in that respect. And associated with this characteristic, I suspect, are a great many social and relational avoidances, whereas with stutterers showing predominantly nonvocalized blocks, the avoidances may be down at a much more specific speech level—at the audibility level, for example.

Dr. Wingate: Already you're beyond the original criterion for discriminating, which, in itself, is not a pure one. That is, you're still faced with the setting-up of criteria for discriminating between certain groups. And even those would be criteria that would still be somewhat questionable—that, you talk about predominantly this or predominantly that.

Dr. Quarrington: The measures need to be sharpened up, but the multidimensionality appears likely.

Dr. Webster: This is a little bit like the problem chemists ran into when they first started differentiating chemistry from alchemy. The question was, what aspect of substances are you concerned with? Color, Smell, Weight, Texture? I think that we probably have to refine our views on stuttered speech, and try to examine more of the details in an effort to determine what features are really salient features and how they relate them to a given set of independent variables which we have available for manipulation.

Dr. Murphy: I think that in terms of the comparative studies that are usually done, on the first part of your question comparing stutterers with nonstutterers, we recognize that while the person who is called stutterer may indeed stutter, the person who is called nonstutterer is usually left in a kind of limbo, unexplained state. And they may, of course, represent a whole variety of disabilities, but as long as they don't stutter, we consider them—what? Normal, probably.

Speaking just a final word or two for myself in terms of the integrity of the syllable, what I'm speaking for is that we don't in our pursuit of the integrity of the syllable lose sight of the integrity of the individual. I personally hope that the emphasis on technique doesn't bring us to the point—as it does in much of our therapy, and this includes not only behavioristic, but a lot of the so-called humanistic therapies, the encounter groups, where technique becomes all pervasive and the central concern of the individual, and the spontaneous wholeness of the individual becomes lost. Technique is important, but not at the expense of individual development. Also to recognize the fact only once more that any technique may be a highly valid technique, but, as Dr. Wingate has illustrated himself, he could not learn as well from an instructor in golf as he could from a book. Now, some people can learn from a book and some people can learn from an instructor. So, in terms of individual differences that we wish to appreciate, not only among persons who stutter, let's appreciate the individual differences that exist among ourselves as clinicians and realize that, while we may be travelling somewhat different pathways, we do have a lot in common in terms of what we want to accomplish. But we do have different ways of doing it. We do have different styles of living. We do have different styles as clinicians. And none ought to be derogated. We ought to look for the qualities of goodness inherent in each one and share them freely.

Dr. Webster: I would like to make one last comment. Our approach is quite technique-oriented. At the same time, it is no less humanistic in its concern for the well-being of the client. It is no less kindly in its treatment of the client than any other form of therapy. I think that it's well to make the point that ours is a warm, person-oriented form of treatment.

Dr. Rieber: That is a very fine note to finish with.

STUTTERING AND QUASI-STUTTERING IN GA

LORRAINE KIRK

Assistant Professor of Anthropology, Department of Sociology and Anthropology,
University of Missouri, St. Louis, Missouri 63121

Introduction

This report is concerned with an unusual stuttering pattern among the Ga. Ga is a tonal language and is a member of the Kwa branch of the Niger-Congo language family. Approximately 700,000 Ga people live in an area of about 500 square miles within and around the city of Accra, Ghana.

The bulk of research on stuttering to date has been done with Indo-European languages; those cross-cultural studies that have been done have dealt primarily with whether or not stuttering is a universal phenomenon (cf. Van Riper, 1971, pp. 4–9). It is of interest to investigate the degree to which stuttering in non-Western languages follows the same patterns found in English. Recent theorists have emphasized that stuttering cannot be understood without reference to the social relationship between speaker and hearer (Johnson, 1959; Sheehan, 1971): stuttering is seen as a consequence of role conflict that produces anxiety in the speaker concerning the production of speech. In the present report Ga stuttering is investigated in terms of (a) the semantic content of the words on which people stutter, (b) the social situations in which people stutter, and (c) the phonological environments of stuttering.

For the purposes of this report, stuttering will be defined as hesitation through either repetition or prolongation of utterance fragments. Stuttering occurs in Ga more frequently than in English or in other European languages with which the author is familiar. Two types of stuttering will be distinguished here on the basis of Ga categories.

The first type of stuttering occurs in very high frequency across both time and individuals. It is hardly perceived by Ga people unless it is clearly demonstrated for them in conversation, in which case they identify it as a thoroughly normal occurrence without particular meaning. They do not seem to have a term for this form of stuttering. The second type of stuttering is intensive and consistent. The Ga recognize this behavior as a pathological syndrome and have a name for it, *háamumɔ,* "to stutter"; *háamuɔlɔ,* *"stutterer."* They often describe a *háamumɔlɔ* as someone who has to force his words out very hard in order to speak, characteristically stamping his foot in his efforts. It is believed that something is wrong with his tongue, and that his difficulties are with him from birth.

The objective of this report is to clarify the nature of stuttering in Ga (a) through a description of social, stylistic, and phonologic factors to which it might be related and (b) through an analysis of its phonologic and semantic distribution.

The materials available for the present analysis of Ga stuttering include (a) field notes taken during 3 months with rural and traditional-urban Ga and (b) approximately 30 hrs. of tapes of rural and traditional-urban Ga verbal behavior recorded in Ghana. The latter do not contain any samples of actual *hámumɔlɔ* speech.

This report consists of two sections: Section I is an ethnographic summary of a series of factors that one might expect to have a causal relation to stuttering. Section II presents the quantitative results of an analysis of the distribution of stuttering by semantic and phonologic context. This analysis is made by comparing the frequencies with which stuttering occurs in various semantic and phonologic contexts to the frequency with which these contexts normally occur in spoken Ga.

I. Ga Interaction and Speech

This section will describe several aspects of the Ga language and culture that may be relevant to the inception of stuttering.

Language Anxiety and Interactional Patterns

Here we shall consider the hypothesis that stuttering in Ga occurs, via tension, as a result of anxiety-provoking circumstances associated with language learning or speech performance. There is evidence in the field notes for the existence of a potentially anxiety-provoking set of experiences surrounding language learning in Ga. The following account is a summary of some aspects of Ga interactional patterns that might contribute to a heightened language anxiety. The observations made here are subjective and therefore tentative, compiled for heuristic purposes only.

The Ga have a reputation among surrounding Ghanaian ethnic groups for roughness. Indeed, they cultivate a strong pretense at toughness, are good with their fists, and are free with threats, insults, and loud, explosive remarks. Although all kinds of violence are exceptionally rare among the Ga, threat and counterthreat are a daily occurrence, both in jest and in seriousness; perhaps this expressive mode makes actual violence less necessary. Children commonly, and adults occasionally, move their bodies and faces in an aggressive way, which might seem to a Westerner to imply a threat of physical attack. Dialogue is generally loud and competitive by United States standards. Parents often direct and reprimand children with intermittent, explosive yells, frequently extending into long loud tirades. Without this tough and threatening presentation, Ga children are not likely to obey. Children themselves display this manner very early (by age two or three), seeking to manage interactions by out-bluffing each other; that is, by putting on a greater show of toughness than their adversaries in the power struggles so frequent among children everywhere. Perhaps the most common verbal threat among both adults and children is an abrupt blast of "I'll beat you!" The freedom to express aggression before a great deal of anger builds up is consistent with the great warmth, humor, and hospitality that are characteristic of the Ga.

Interruptions also seem from a United States perspective to be strikingly sharp and frequent in Ga conversation. People interrupt by speaking very loudly and drowning out the speaker or by suddenly refocusing the listener's attention. The speaker may then finish his word to thin air or stop in the middle of the word. The groups within which conversation normally takes place are generally larger in Ga than in United States homes, and this may tend to increase the number of interruptions that occur. Under these circumstances it often seems difficult for small children to make themselves heard.

It is my impression that there is more of an emphasis on form than on content in much of rural and traditional-urban Ga verbal interaction. Speech prowess does not seem to be judged so much in terms of subject matter or factual content as in terms of eloquence of pronunciation, loudness, forcefulness, rhythm, adeptness in the selection of words, and ability to remember and work into the conversation traditional verbal seuqences. In answering factual questions as well there appears to be a deemphasis on specific content. Children ask questions, but adults often seem to consider it unimportant either that the child know the answer or that he be given a direct answer. Adults more often than not either brush off the question, change the subject, or give an answer that does not seem to deal with the content of the question.

Speech activity as such is strongly encouraged in both adults and children, as well as in interested foreigners. Adults listen and respond to children especially when they perform traditional forms or songs, either alone or in groups. But it is the recitation itself, not so much the semantic content of the words, that appears to be enjoyed. Speech encouragement is, further, highly directive.[1] One very frequently hears adults or older children telling small children to "say _____" or taking the words out of their mouths. Adults and older children correct the speech of younger people in traditional forms. Sometimes they continue the recitation when the corrected child stops. For my tape recorder children were often encouraged to speak, but through loud, abrupt shouts of "Speak! Speak!" This more often than not frightened the children into rigid silence.

---

[1]Perhaps some of this description is biased more than I know by the fact that sometimes children were being encouraged to speak for me.

Some amount of oral threat is observable in the way in which small children are teased with "You won't eat anymore!" This is sometimes used for disciplinary purposes, sometimes as teasing. Crying frequently follows, after which the threat is withdrawn, as, for example, with "You will eat; you will eat yams," and the crying stops.

Stylistic and Phonologic Considerations

There are alternatives to the hypothesis that the widespread "normal" stuttering of the Ga is conditioned by threatening influences associated with language. It might be suggested that stuttering in Ga is a stylistic way of laying emphasis. People in Ga seem to emphasize points by speaking more explosively than usual. This contrasts with the tendency for speakers of English to be emphatic through clearer enunciation and changes in tone and phoneme length, with only minimal changes in volume. An informant from Fanti, an ethnic group neighboring the Ga, has described the Ga language as more threatening, forceful, and aggressive than Fanti, and has suggested that stuttering should be found especially in aggressive and abusive behavior.

Finally, the phonologic nature of the Ga language itself may be relevant to an understanding of the stuttering observed. Ga words are short, characteristically beginning with a highly explosive consonant cluster and ending with a short, clipped vowel. A great proportion of words in common use consist of one syllable only. It is not possible to ease into the pronunciation of a word as in English, French, or even German. Phonology may also therefore be postulated to account for some of the jerky repetition of speech fragments so common in Ga. Alternatively, the phonologic nature of the language may make stuttering more obvious when it does occur.

II. Analysis of Taped Materials

This section will analyze data from the tapes of Ga speech. These data will be limited to "normal" stuttering in lieu of tapes on *háamumɔlɔ* speech. Approximately 30 hrs. of tapes of Ga verbal behavior are examined for repetition or prolongation of utterance fragments, together with information on the affected utterance, the identity of the speaker, and the social context. Repeated or prolongated utterance fragments are tabulated only where clear enough to be transcribed. Repetitions of complete utterances are excluded, as well as hesitations consisting of substitutions of a new word for that already begun.

The tapes of verbal behavior were collected in a Ga village over a period of 3 months. The tape recorder was set up near people at work, at play, and in conversational groups. Large and small group interactions were both well represented. Speakers ranged in age from 2½ to elder; both sexes were represented among young children, older children, adults, and elders. All speakers were personally known to the author; none had exhibited the pattern of behavior characteristic of pathological or abnormal stutterers (*háamumɔlɔi*).

The questions asked of the resulting data are restricted by a number of problems that arose during the collection of data from the tapes. A prime obstacle in transcribing the environments of stutterers is the unusual jerkiness and imprecision that, it became apparent, characterize the environments of stuttering. This is confounded by the fact that a high proportion of stuttering occurs in large group situations, with much interruption and overlapping speech. The net effect is that utterances in which repetitions of speech fragments occur are some of the hardest to transcribe and understand. This leads to gaps in the data. Where data are scarce or garbled on a particular question, only the clear data are tabulated, resulting in different sample sizes for each analysis.

Quantitative Results

Position of beginning of repeated or prolonged utterance fragment in word. Tables 1 and 2 demonstrate that stuttering occurs much more frequently

TABLE 1
Position of Beginning of Repeated or Prolonged Fragment in Word

A.   Assuming that personal pronouns and possessives constitute words separate from the verb

Position in word	Number of occurrences of stuttering
Initial	197
Middle	4
Final	0
Indeterminate	26

B.   Assuming that personal pronoun or possessive in combination with the verb constitutes a word

Position in word	Number of occurrences of stuttering
Initial	195
Middle	6
Final	0
Indeterminate	26

TABLE 2
Position in Word Cross-Tabulated with Repetition or Prolongation

	Initial position	Other
Repeated or prolongated fragments	197	4
Independent sample of speech	417	304

Chi square = 192.3 (df = 1).
$P < 0.0005$.

(approximately 95% of the time) at the beginnings of words than would be predicted by chance. There are 197 cases of stuttering at word beginnings, 4 cases of stuttering at other positions in words, and 26 cases in which the positions in words could not be determined. By contrast, in an independent sample of Ga speech, there are 417 phonemes in initial positions of words and 304 phonemes in other positions. The chi-square value for this comparison is 192.3 ($P < 0.0005$). This result is consistent with findings from English. Von Riper (1971, p. 188)

TABLE 3A
Fragments Repeated or Prolongated

Fragment	f	Fragment	f
a	28	ʔ	4
ay	2	y	4
amɛ	3	ye	1
atʃɔ̃	1	ya	1
aba	1	kɔ	2
abanyɛ	1	ka	1
e	25	kwɛ	1
ee	1	kwɛ o	1
ɛ	5	kɛ	2
ekɛn	1	kɛɛ	1
ew	1	k	2
èbé	1	b	2
ɛ̀bɛ́	1	ba	3
élè	1	bibio	1
eŋɔɔ	1	bɛ	1
m	21	bo	1
ma	8	g	2
mi	3	Gã	1
mika	1	gbɛ	1
ʌm	1	t	1
mɛ	3	tʃ wanõ	1
mɛni	3	l	2
n	15	la	1
ny	2	lɛ	1
ŋ	6	dz (= ǰ)	1
ŋkɛɛ	2	d	1
ŋla	1	ɔ	1
ŋgbɛ	1	hã	1
o	16	i	1
ok	1		209
odz (= oǰ)	1		
oba	1		
wɔ	5		
wɔʃĩ	1		
wa	1		

TABLE 3B
Fragments Repeated or Prolongated, Summary A

Personal pronouns and possessives:	f	Other	f
m (in contracted 1st person sing.):		m	10
Present tense (mi)	3	m + following segment	6
Future tense (ma)	8		
mi (1st person singular)	3		
mi (1st person singular + following segment)	1		
m (contracted 1st person singular possessive)	1		
ma (contracted 1st person singular future)	8		
ŋ (contracted 1st person sing.		ŋ	1
present and contracted 1st			
person sing. possessive)	6		
ŋ (above + following segment)	3		
o (2nd person singular)	16		
o (2nd person singular + following segment)	3		
lɛ (3rd person singular)	1	l	3
e (3rd person singular)	26		
e (3rd person singular + following segment)	6		
ɛ (3rd person singular)	5		
wɔ (1st person plural)	5	wa	1
wɔ (1st person plural + following segment)	1		
n (in nyɛ = 2nd person plural)	2	n	13
nyɛ (2nd person plural)	2		
a (3rd person plural)	28		
a (3rd person plural + following segment)	8		
	136	k	10
		b	8
		y	6
		g	4
		ʔ	4
		t	2
		d	1
		dz (= ǰ)	1
		h	1
		ɔ	1
		i	1
			73

states, "All investigators have found that more stuttering occurs on initial sounds or syllables than on later sounds or syllables."

Preponderance of stuttering on personal pronouns or possessives. Table 3A lists stuttered utterance fragments transcribed from the tape, together with the frequency with which the fragments are stuttered. Only fragments clear enough on tape to be reliably transcribed are included. Where an utterance with a repeated or prolongated fragment is pronounced two or more times in succession with identical repetition or prolongation, only one sample from the series is transcribed and tabulated in Table 3A.

Tables 3B and 3C summarize the data of Table 3A. Table 3B regroups repeated and prolongated fragments in a way that demonstrates that the occurrence of stuttering on personal pronouns or possessives is approximately twice as frequent as stuttering on all other forms combined. One hundred and thirty-six out of 209 cases of stuttering are on personal pronouns or possessives (65.1%). In a sample of speech from the stuttered corpus, personal pronouns and possessives total 61 out of 205 lexical items (29.8%). In an independent sample of Ga speech, personal

TABLE 3C
Fragments Repeated or Prolongated, Summary B

Stuttering begins with	f
Consonants	
Nasal continuants	
m	40
n	17
	10
Other consonants	
k	10
b	8
w	7
y	6
g	4
l	4
ʔ	4
t	1
tʃ	1
dz (= ǰ)	1
d	1
h	1
	115
Vowels	
a	36
e	32
o	19
ɛ	5
ɔ	1
i	1
	94

TABLE 4A
Personal Pronouns and Possessives Cross-Tabulated with Repetition or Prolongation: Comparison with Stuttered Corpus

	Personal pronouns and possessives	Other
Repeated or prolongated fragments	136	73
Sample of speech from stuttered corpus	61	144

Chi square = 51.8 (df = 1).
P < 0.0005.

pronouns and possessives constitute 180 out of 811 lexical items (22.2%). Chi-square tests on these two contrasts (Tables 4A and 4B) are highly significant [51.8 and 142.9, respectively (P < 0.0005)]. The high frequency of Ga stuttering on personal pronouns and possessives is parallel to Bloodstein and Gantwerk's (1967) finding of high frequency stuttering on personal pronouns and conjunctions, and is consistent with Sheehan's hypothesis (1970) that stuttering is a consequence of role conflict. Sheehan notes a tendency to stutter on the personal pronoun "I."

A possible interpretation of these findings is that the relevant variable is reference to persons as such; this tends to support the hypotheses that stuttering is related to language anxiety, and that this anxiety is highly associated with social relationship. However, two cautions should be noted about the present data. The first is that only an additional six repetitions or prolongations of person names, specific and classificatory, are found in the total corpus. The second caution is that "personal pronouns" here include "it" as well as persons, as "he," "she," and "it" are indistinguishable in Ga apart from context. Sometimes distant context is necessary to make a distinction, and frequently the relevant context is not on the tape. Hence a reliable breakdown of personal pronouns and possessives in terms of persons as opposed to things is not feasible.

Types of phonemes on which stuttering occurs. Table 3C also summarizes the data of Table 3A, showing frequency of occurrence of vowels and consonants.

TABLE 4B

Personal Pronouns and Possessives Cross-Tabulated with Repetition or Prolongation: Comparison with Independent Corpus

	Personal pronouns and possessives	Other
Repeated or prolonged fragments	136	73
Independent sample of speech	180	631

Chi square = 142.9 (df = 1).
P < 0.0005.

TABLE 5A

Contrast among Vowels, Nasal Continuants, and Other Consonants Cross-Tabulated with Repetition or Prolongation

	Vowels	Nasal continuants	Other Consonants	
Repeated or prolonged fragments	94 (70.5)[a]	67 (48.7)	48 (89.8)	209
Independent sample of speech	203 (226.5)	138 (156.3)	330 (288.2)	671
	297	205	378	880

Chi square = 44.79 (df = 2).
P < 0.0005.
[a] Expected values in parentheses.

TABLE 5B
Contrast between Vowels and Nasal Continuants Cross-Tabulated with Repetition or Prolongation

	Vowels	Nasal continuants	
Repeated or prolongated fragments	94	67	161
Independent sample of speech	203	138	341
	297	205	502

Chi square = 0.06 (NS).

TABLE 6
Personal Pronouns and Possessives Cross-Tabulated with Vowels and Nasal Continuants in Initial
Positions of Words

	Personal pronouns and possessives	Other lexical items
Vowels and nasal continuants	109	172
Other consonants	17	239

Chi square = 77.1 (df = 1).
$P < 0.0005$.

From the table it can be seen that 94 stuttering blocks occur on vowels, 67 on nasal continuants (*m, n,* and *ŋ*), and 48 on other consonants. By contrast (Table 5A), in an independent sample of word beginnings[2] in Ga speech, vowels occur 203 times, nasal continuants 138 times, and other consonants 330 times. These data indicate that the incidence of stuttering is much higher for vowels and nasal continuants than it is for other consonants (chi square = 44.79; $P < 0.0005$). This effect is no doubt related to the fact that most personal pronouns and possessives used in rapid Ga speech begin with either vowels or nasal continuants.

If we look at the occurrence of vowels versus nasal continuants (Table 5B), we see that 94 stuttering blocks occur on vowels, while 67 occur on nasal continuants. By contrast, our independent sample of word beginnings from Ga speech shows an occurrence of 203 vowels and 138 nasal continuants. In the stuttered corpus, vowels are 58.4% of the total; in the control, 59.5% of the total. The chi-square value is 0.06. These figures show no difference between vowels and nasal continuants in the frequency with which they are stuttered in the corpus.

It is of interest here to ask whether the high frequency of stuttering on vowels and nasal continuants is due to the tendency to stutter on personal pronouns, or vice versa. In a sample of Ga word beginnings independent of the stuttering corpus, 109 personal pronouns or possessives begin with vowels or nasal continuants and 17 begin with other consonants (Table 6). Of the lexical items at word beginnings other than personal pronouns and possessives, 172 begin with vowels or nasal continuants and 239 begin with other consonants. The chi-square value is 77.1 for

---

[2]Phonemes at word beginnings were selected as a subsample of Ga phonemes because of our earlier observation that most stuttering occurs at the beginnings of words.

TABLE 7

Contrast among Nasal Continuants, Vowels, and Other Consonants Outside of Personal Pronouns and Possessives, Cross-Tabulated with Repetition or Prolongation

	Nasal continuants	Vowels	Other consonants	
Repeated or prolongated fragments outside of personal pronouns or possessives	30 (15.7)[a]	2 (19.1)	37 (34.21)	69
Independent sample of speech	138 (152.3)	203 (185.9)	330 (332.8)	671
	168	205	367	740

Chi square = 31.7 (df = 2).
$P < 0.0005$.
[a] Expected values in parentheses.

TABLE 8
Preceding Environment

Phoneme	f
Pause	117
a	21
ã	1
ɛ	10
ɛ̃	2
e	9
i	9
ī	3
o	3
ɔ	1
ɔ̃	1
ū	1
Summary	
Nasal	8
Non-nasal	53
a + ã	22 (low central unrounded)
e + ɛ + ɛ̃	21 (mid front unrounded)
i + ī	12 (high front unrounded)
o	3 (mid back rounded)
ɔ + ɔ̃	2 (low back rounded)
ū	1 (high back rounded)
Unrounded	55
Rounded	6
Front	33
Central	22
Back	6
Low	24
Mid	24
High	13

this comparison ($P < 0.0005$), showing that personal pronouns/possessives begin with vowels and nasals in very high frequency (87%).

Controlling for the effects of the frequency with which stuttering occurs on personal pronouns or possessives by looking only at stuttering on lexical items other than personal pronouns and possessives, we see from Table 7 that 30 cases of stuttering occur on nasal continuants, 2 on vowels, and 37 on other consonants. In our independent sample of word beginnings from Ga speech, 138 words begin with nasal continuants, 203 words begin with vowels, and 330 words begin with other consonants. We can see from Table 7 that among stuttering not occurring on personal pronouns or possessives there is a strong tendency to stutter on nasal continuants and an equally strong tendency not to stutter on vowels. This is consistent with Hahn's (1942) finding that only 2.9% of stuttering occurred on words beginning with vowels. Similarly Brown (1938) found more stuttering on consonants than on vowels.

It can be concluded that the observed tendency to stutter on vowels or nasal continuants has two causes: (a) the tendency to stutter on personal pronouns or possessives, which usually begin with vowels (see Table 3B) and (b) the tendency for stuttering not occurring on personal pronouns or possessives to begin with nasals. The tendency to stutter on nasals is obscured in the sample, as there is a strong tendency to stutter on personal pronouns or possessives, which do not usually begin with nasal continuants (see Table 3B).

Preceding environment. The environment immediately preceding repeated or prolongated fragments is tabulated in Table 8. It is evident from the table that a large number of repetitions and prolongations occur at the beginnings of utterances or phrases, or after pauses (117 out of 178 stutters occur following pauses). From the table it is also clear that stuttering consistently follows vowels. This may be an artifact of a combination of two factors: (a) most stuttering blocks begin where words begin (Table 1) and (b) most Ga words end with vowels.

From the summary of Table 8 it can also be seen that preceding vowels are predominantly unrounded rather than rounded, and front rather than back. In environments immediately preceding stuttering blocks, there are 55 cases of unrounded vowels and 6 cases of rounded vowels, while in an independent sample of Ga speech unrounded vowels occur 385 times and rounded vowels 151 times (Table 9). The chi-square value is 9.5 ($P < 0.005$). In environments immediately preceding stuttering there are 33 cases of front vowels and 6 cases of back vowels,

TABLE 9

Preceding Environment: Contrast between Unrounded and Rounded Vowels Cross-Tabulated with Repetition or Prolongation

	Unrounded vowels	Rounded vowels
Repeated or prolonged fragments	55	6
Independent sample of speech	385	151

Chi square = 9.5 ($df = 1$).
$P < 0.005$.

TABLE 10
Preceding Environment: Contrast between Front and Back Vowels Cross-Tabulated with Repetition or Prolongation

	Front vowels	Back vowels
Repeated or prolongated fragments	33	6
Independent sample of speech	292	151

Chi square = 4.3 (df = 1).
P < 0.05.

TABLE 11
Following Environment

Vowels	f	Consonants	f
a	26	n	16
ɛ	12	b	13
e	7	k	11
i	5	h	10
o	5	tʃ (= č)	9
ɔ	5	m	9
u	1	y	8
	61	+ or #	6
		dz (=ǰ)	6
		t	5
		w̆	5
		f	4
		l	3
		ʃ (= š)	3
		g	2
		d	1
		η	1
		s	1
			113

TABLE 12
Following Environment: Contrast between Consonants and Vowels Cross-Tabulated with Repetition or Prolongation

	Consonants	Vowels
Repeated or prolongated fragments	113	61
Independent sample of speech	428	562

Chi square = 28.0 (df = 1).
P < 0.0005.

while in an independent speech sample, front vowels occur 292 times and back vowels 151 times (Table 10). The chi-square value here is 4.3 ($P < 0.05$). With the exception of the vowel *a*, which is central and unrounded, the front-back distinction is identical to the rounded-unrounded distinction in Ga (Fig. 1, p. 122).

Following environment. Table 11 shows the frequency with which each phoneme follows repeated or prolonged fragments. In Tables 11 and 12 we see that consonants occur almost twice as frequently as vowels in positions immediately following repeated or prolonged fragments (there are 113 consonants out of

	Front		Central		Back	
	Unrounded	Rounded	Unrounded	Rounded	Unrounded	Rounded
High	i					u
Mid	e ɛ					o ɔ
Low			a			

Fig. 1. Ga vowels.

174 phonemes following stuttered utterance fragments). In an independent sample of speech, consonants occur 428 times and vowels 562 times (chi square = 28.0, P < 0.0005).

Number of hesitations per repeated fragment. Table 13 distinguishes between repetitions and single prolongations, with prolongations simultaneous with repetitions counted here as repetitions. On this basis, the table indicates that mean number of repetitions per repeated fragment is 2.89 (i.e., the fragment is pronounced 2.89 times on the average), with a consistent decrease in frequency of occurrence with increased number of repetitions per fragment. It also shows that a single prolongation without actual repetition is less frequent than a double or triple repetition (fragment pronounced 2 or 3 times), but more common than a repetition of 4 or greater.

Competition, speaker, and frequency of personal pronouns and possessives with three or more repetitions per stutter. Table 14 compares stuttering of high intensity (involving three or more repetitions per utterance fragment) with less intensive stutterers (involving one or two repetitions per fragment). Comparisons are made of frequencies of (a) competitive context,[3] (b) stuttering on personal pronouns or possessives, (c) adult and adolescent male speaker as opposed to all other types of speaker, and (d) adolescent male speaker as opposed to adult male speaker. Tables 14 through 18 show that when we examine only stuttering involving three or more repetitions per fragment, to the exclusion of stuttering involving one or two repetitions per fragment, (a) evidence of competition is greater (chi square = 11.8, P < 0.001), (b) proportion of personal pronouns and possessives among repeated fragments is greater (chi square = 4.7, P < 0.05), (c) proportions of stuttering by adult and adolescent males to stuttering by all others is

---

[3] Contextual situations in which stuttering occurred were divided into two categories for the purpose of this measurement: those in which more than normal competition would be expected to be present and those in which there was no evidence by which to classify the situation as competitive. In making these judgments, a series of factors were considered, such as the number of people present in the interaction, whether there was fighting or arguing, and the occurrence of overt interruption of the speaker. One hundred and twenty-two cases of stuttering occurred under what appears to be the pressure of competition, while the remaining 74 cases could not be judged to have occurred in competitive situations.

TABLE 13
Number of Hesitations per Repeated Fragment

Number of repetitions	f
2	104
3	42
4	21
5	12
6	5
7	3
8	1
9	0
10	1
Single prolongation only	34

Average number of repetitions per fragment = 2.89

Distribution of single prolongations	
2½-year-old female	28
Adolescent male	2
Adult male	4
	34

TABLE 14
Competition, Speaker, and Frequency of Personal Pronouns and Possessives with Three or More Repetitions per Fragment

	Number of stuttering blocks with three or more repetitions per fragment
Competition	
Judged present	58
Not assessed	17
Personal pronouns and possessives	
Stuttering occurs on personal pronoun or possessive	56
Stuttering occurs on other form	19
Speaker	
Adult male	31
Adolescent male	26
Male child	6
Female child	7
Adult female	5

TABLE 15
Judged Presence of Competition Cross-Tabulated with Intensity of Stuttering

	Stuttering with three or more repetitions	Stuttering with one or two repetitions
Competition judged present	58	64
Competition undetermined	17	57

Chi square = 11.8 (df = 1).
$P < 0.001$.

TABLE 16
Personal Pronouns and Possessives Cross-Tabulated with Intensity of Stuttering

	Stuttering with three or more repetitions	Stuttering with one or two repetitions
Personal pronouns or possessives	56	80
Other forms	19	54

Chi square = 4.7 (df = 1).
$P < .05$.

TABLE 17
Speaker: Contrast between Post-pubescent Males and All Others Cross-Tabulated with Intensity of Stuttering

	Stuttering with three or more repetitions	Stuttering with one or two repetitions
Males past puberty	57	65
Others	18	60

Chi square = 11.3 (df = 1).
$P < 0.001$.

TABLE 18
Speaker: Contrast between Adolescent Males and Adult Males Cross-Tabulated with Intensity of Stuttering

	Stuttering with three or more repetitions	Stuttering with one or two repetitions
Adolescent males	26	21
Adult males	31	44

Chi square = 2.3 (df = 1).
$P < 0.20$.

greater (chi square = 11.3, $P < 0.001$), and (d) proportion of stuttering by adolescent males to stuttering by adult males is slightly greater (chi square = 2.3, $P < 0.20$). It may be tentatively concluded that (a) greater competition is associated with more intensive stuttering, (b) personal pronouns and possessives are more clearly selected fragments for repetition in more intensive stutterers than in less intensive stutterers, and (c) post-puberty males in general, and adolescent males specifically, have more of a monopoly on more intense stuttering than they do on less intense stuttering. These findings are consistent with findings of Sheehan (1970) and Schuell (1946, 1947). Sheehan hypothesizes that stuttering is a consequence of role conflict, and finds that people stutter more in conversation with higher status people. Schuell reports that males stutter much more than females.

Conclusions

An unusual stuttering pattern has been observed in Ga. This report has approached the phenomenon from two perspectives.

First, ethnographic materials that might be related to Ga stuttering have been presented as evidence for alternate interpretations of the stuttering as a function of (a) language anxiety, (b) style, and (c) phonologic factors. All three interpretations are offered as plausible.

Second, an empirical study of several samples of Ga speech has been undertaken. The speech samples include utterances in which "ordinary," nonpathological stuttering occurs. These samples have been analyzed, comparing the distribution of stuttered utterance fragments to the distribution of utterance fragments in random samples of Ga speech. Variables pertaining to the social identity of the speaker, the social context, and the semantics and phonology of stuttered fragments and their immediate environments have been considered in this analysis. With respect to nonpathological stuttering, a series of conclusions might be drawn:

1. Stuttering occurs predominantly (about 95% of the time) in the initial positions of words, and almost half the stuttering occurs in the beginnings of utterances, clauses, or phrases.

2. A preponderance of the stuttering occurs on personal pronouns or possessives, possibly indicating a high frequency of stuttering in reference to persons.

3. There is a strong tendency to stutter on nasal continuants. This effect is independent of the above tendency to stutter on personal pronouns or possessives.

4. All stuttering not following + or # follow vowels. Consonants do not occur prior to stuttering.

5. Vowels preceding stuttering are predominantly unrounded and front.

6. The occurrence of vowels in positions following stuttering is rare relative to their occurrence in Ga speech.

7. Vowels are proportionately most frequent in contrast with consonants immediately prior to stuttering, least frequent immediately following stuttering, and of intermediate frequency in initial positions of stuttering.

8. A much broader distribution of phonemes can be seen in positions immediately following stuttering than in positions immediately prior to stuttering. This may indicate that there is less selection occurring in the placement of stuttering in terms of following environment than of prior environment, or it may be to some extent an artifact of the fact that stuttering blocks vary in the numbers of phonemes that they incorporate.

9. Repeated utterance fragments are pronounced an average of 2.89 times. Stuttering decreases in frequency with increased number of repetitions per fragment. A single prolongation without repetition has a frequency of occurrence intermediate between those for three and four repetitions.

10. In considering more intensive stuttering alone, certain tendencies observed for stutters in general are seen to be intensified.

11. Greater competition is associated with more intensive stuttering.

12. Personal pronouns and possessives are yet more clearly selected as fragments for repetition in more intensive (repetitive) stuttering than in stuttering in general.

Summary

This report considers two types of stuttering in Ga. Language anxiety, style, and phonologic and semantic factors have been offered as plausible sources of stuttering. These have been considered through some ethnographic remarks and through an analysis of the occurrence of the more frequent, nonpathological form of stuttering in Ga.

Repetition or prolongation of utterance fragments is shown to occur predominantly on personal pronouns or possessives. It is proposed that a relevant variable here may be reference to persons, stuttering being encouraged by language anxiety associated with social relationship.

Several other observations have been made about the distribution of nonpathological stuttering in Ga. Repetitions and prolongations of utterance fragments almost always occur at the beginnings of words. All of the phonemes immediately preceding stuttering are vowels. The phonemes immediately following stuttering tend to be consonants; however, there is more variation in the following environment than in the preceding environment. Finally, stronger results are obtained in some cases when only the more intensive stutters are considered than when all intensities of stuttering are considered together.

Two questions remain to be answered: (a) How universal cross-culturally are the stuttering patterns that we have observed in the Ga language? and (b) Do the pathological and nonpathological forms of stuttering in Ga differ only in intensity or are they qualitatively distinct as well? Hence it would be useful to compare the present data with stuttering patterns in other languages and with the pathological pattern of stuttering in Ga.

References

Bloodstein, O., Gantwerk, B. F. Grammatical function in relation to stuttering in young children. *J. Speech Hearing Res.*, 1967, **10**, 786–89.

Brown, S. F. Stuttering with relation to word accent and word position. *J. Abnorm. Soc. Psychol.*, 1938, **33**, 112–120.

Hahn, E. A study of the relationship between stuttering occurrence and phonetic factors in oral reading. *J. Speech Dis.*, 1942, **7**, 143–151.

Johnson, W. *The onset of stuttering: research findings and implications.* Minneapolis: University of Minnesota Press, 1959.

Schuell, H. Sex differences in relation to stuttering, Part I. *J. Speech Dis.*, 1946, **11**, 277–298.

Schuell, H. Sex differences in relation to stuttering, Part II. *J. Speech Dis.*, 1947, **12**, 23–28.

Sheehan, J. G., (Ed.). *Stuttering: research and therapy.* New York: Harper & Row, 1970.

Van Riper, C. *The nature of stuttering.* Englewood Cliffs, N. J.: Prentice-Hall, 1971.

HIERONYMUS MERCURIALIS

Treatises on the Diseases of Children, most copious, and filled with diverse doctrine, highly useful not only to physicians, but indeed to philosophers as well; diligently taken down from the mouth of the most excellent, most famous physician Hieronymus Mercurialis of Forli, by the labors of Johannes Chrosczieyoioskius.

Translator's Note: As explained in the introduction to this book, the word *balbutiēs*, although its meaning certainly includes the problem of stuttering, does not really correspond to any currently recognized clinical entity. For this reason, and to avoid further ambiguity, it has been thought best to leave the words *balbutiēs* (the state or quality of being *balbus*) and *balbus* (affected with *balbutiēs*, a person so affected) untranslated. Mercurialis' usage of these words is clearly explained in a passage from Book 2, Chapter 6 ("On Speech Defects in General"), which we have printed below, immediately preceding the complete Chapter 8 ("On *Balbutiēs*"). The text used in the present translation is that of the Basel 1584 edition. Much advantage was derived from comparison with an earlier translation by Dr. Herbert F. Wright, in John Ruhrah, ed., *Pediatrics of the Past* (New York, 1925), pp. 225–236. Nevertheless, it was felt that this previous version had not entirely done justice to the Latin text, which, austere in style, requires for that very reason a greater effort not only to render it with accuracy and clarity, but also to preserve what little style it has.

Editorial interpolations are in brackets [ ].

JEFFREY WOLLOCK

Section on the History of Psychiatry and the Behavioral Sciences, Cornell Univ. Medical College, 525 East 68th Street, New York, NY 10019

[After distinguishing muteness as a first kind of defect, Mercurialis continues with the following (based largely on Aristotle, *Problems xi.30*)]: . . . "If speech should occur with difficulty, another kind of defect arises, which in Aëtius is called *mogilalia*; we can call it an *impediment of speech*. If the speech should be disfigured, a third kind of defect occurs, referred to by Hippocrates *(Aphorisms vi.32)* under the generic name of *traulotes,* or *traulosis*: we also call it by the generic name of *balbutiēs*.

"Of this last defect, moreover, I find three kinds in the literature. The first is when speech cannot be uttered at once, when a man or a child is compelled to repeat the first or some other syllable of a word with great effort. A defect of this sort is called by Hippocrates and Aristotle *ischnophonia*; some of the Latin writers refer to it as a "staggering of the tongue" *(titubantia linguae)*, but that most learned Theodore of Gaza best of all calls it a "hesitating of the tongue" *(haesitans linguae)*. I also find that this defect has been called *batarismus*, after Batarus,[1] king of the Cyrenes, who was always forced to repeat the first syllable of a word.

"Another defect, or type of *balbutiēs*, is when a child omits some syllable, that is, when he is completely unable to pronounce a word or name in full. Galen, and with him all others, calls this *pselloteta*.[2] Aristotle refers to those suffering under this kind of affection as *blaesi*. . . .

"A third type of *balbutiēs* is that called (in common with some other defects) *traulotes*, and this, as Galen writes in his 6th commentary to the *Aphorisms* of Hippocrates, Ch. 32, is when a man or child cannot produce an r, but changes it to l . . . this category also includes the change from c to t[3] . . . and this third type of *balbutiēs* has been commemorated as the affliction of Demosthenes and Alcibiades. . . ." [Thus, wherever the words *balbutiēs* and *balbus* (plural *balbi*) appear in what follows, unless further qualified, they should be taken as referring generically to all these defects.]

Book 2, Chapter 8: *On Balbutiēs*

We proceed to the impediment of speech, either *mogilalia* or *ankyloglossia*. This affection has two causes: one native, the other accidental and by disease. A native cause, as Galen teaches, *On the Use of the Parts xi. 10*, is an unnatural attachment of the tongue with the underlying parts, which very often happens in children; a cause which is certainly by disease, is either a tumor beneath the tongue, as in *ranula*, or a scar left by a wound of that part. The causes which have been proposed were also related by Aëtius[4] in such a way as to include no others.

---

[1]*Sic* for Battus. See Herodotus iv. 155.

[2]I am not aware of any use of precisely this word by Galen, although *psellidzesthai*, which presumably means the same thing, is found in his commentary to *Aphorism 6.32*, *psellidzein* in his 3rd commentary to Hippocrates' 1st book of *Predications*, and *pselloi* (those affected with *psellismos*) in *De Locīs Affecīīs 4.9*. In none of these, however, does Galen define any further than to specify that it is a defect of speech rather than of voice. But in his commentary 6 to the 2nd book of *Epidemics*, he says, contrary to the assertion of Mercurialis, that *psellos* denotes *one who corrupts the S*. (The Greek original of this book of commentaries disappeared in the early Middle Ages, and was virtually unknown in Europe, surviving only in the Arabic translation of Hunain ibn Ishaq. It was translated into German only as recently as 1934 by E. Wenkebach and F. Pfaff.)

[3]Not in Galen; it is, however, mentioned in Quintilian, I. xi. 6.

[4]*Tetrabiblos*, Bk. II, Serm. iv, Ch. 36.

Now follows the third defect, which is *balbutiēs*, or disfigured speech. Although this consists of three types, the cause of each one pertains to an injury either of faculty or of instruments. The faculty is injured when either the brain itself is disturbed by some distemper,[5] or when the faculty itself is held back in its ability to run across and move the tongue correctly. A distemper of the brain occurs in drunkenness, for Galen said, *Aphorisms vi.32,* that drunkards are *balbi* because the brain is more moist than it should be, and consequently along with it the instruments moving the tongue, as well as the tongue itself. A distemper of the brain also occurs in frenzy,[6] in which, since the brain has been heated and dried out, the imaginative faculty cannot work effectively to move the tongue as it should.

Moreover the faculty is detained from its function in ecstasy, and in melancholy. In ecstasy certainly, because, distracted by phantasms, it by no means governs the tongue as it ought. In melancholy, it is impeded by three causes: one is fear, which is melancholy's constant companion, and hence Aristotle, *Problems xi.36*[7] said that when in fear, people become *balbi*. And this is also what Hippocrates said, *2 Epidemics vi.1,* where he wrote that *balbi* become melancholy.[8]

The imagination, or its faculty,[9] is impeded in a second way in melancholy: because it is moved very forcefully. This proposition is handed down by Aëtius,[10] in accordance with an opinion of Ruffus and Posidonius, and certainly it does happen that by great motion the imagination wanders, and also on account of this wandering, that it does not properly control the tongue. And this is what Hippocrates said in his *Book of Precepts,* that the tongue is often *balbus* from a wandering of the mind.

A third cause is multitude of phantasms and imaginations. For Aristotle, *Problems xi.38,* expounding the cause of hesitation of the tongue, seems among other things to place variety and multitude of imaginations, because, as long as the faculty is pursuing this or that phantasm, the tongue cannot diligently follow the action of the faculty at all. Hence it wanders, and hesitancy occurs. And these are the kinds of causes which pertain to the faculty itself, as far as concerns *balbutiēs*.

Certainly the causes pertaining to the instruments are either natural defects, or preternatural; or, as Galen put it, *On the Affected Parts iv.9,* they occur either in

---

[5]I.e., a disturbance of the balance of the four humors by the overproduction of one.

[6]I. e., phrenitis, inflamation of the brain.

[7]All references to this work have been adjusted to correspond with the numbering in the edition of W. S. Hett (Cambridge: Loeb series, 1939).

[8]This passage of Hippocrates is very obscure and is read differently by different editors.

[9]The faculty of forming images in the mind, considered to be the basis of all thought.

[10]*Tetrabiblos,* Bk. II, Serm. ii, Ch. 9.

the very formation of the instruments, or after their formation. Of whichever kind the defects may be, however, their causes are either similar to disease, or instrumental.

Those which are similar to disease are, in particular, cold and moist distempers, sometimes of the tongue itself, but most of all of the muscles moving the tongue and larynx. This is what Galen, *1 Epidemics ii.78,* wished to signify when he wrote that *ischnophonia* occurs from a feebleness of the muscles of the larynx, caused by a lessening of heat.[11] And it is what Aristotle, *Problems xi. 10, 30, 36,* showed us, before Galen, when he wrote that *balbuties* and hesitancy of tongue occur from cold and moisture.

But touching this opinion a doubt arises, that is, whether *balbuties* occurs *only* by a cold and moist distemper; for Galen, *Aphorisms vi.32,* says that every *balbuties* which has been suffered seems related to moisture; nay, he actually writes that *balbuties* in children can never arise from dryness. This seems also to be what *Aristotle, xi.30,* meant to convey, when he said that more children than men are *balbi,* that is, on account of their moisture. But to the contrary is Hippocrates, *7 Epidemics 2 and 3,* where, narrating the history of certain people who were ill, he says that they had a somewhat *balbus* tongue[12] on account of dryness. From this passage one plainly gathers that *balbuties* also occurs on account of dryness. Avicenna, *Canon iii fen 6.3.16,* manifestly says the same.

By way of reconciling the disagreement of these authorities, it must be said that *balbuties* is of two kinds, one natural, the other accidental. The natural occurs in no other way than that proposed by Galen, namely, from moisture. But the unnatural, that is, the accidental, can likewise occur from dryness; and it is of this that Hippocrates and Avicenna spoke.

Moreover the manner in which natural moisture causes *balbuties,* and why it happens that some people are unable to pronounce r, or c, is that for their pronunciation it is necessary that the tongue be strongly impelled against the teeth and palate. A tongue which is soft, however, or too moist, or is feeble on account of the moisture of its muscles, cannot be impelled toward the teeth as forcefully as it should. Hence in place of this letter others are pronounced which, although similar, do not require so great an impulse.[13] We can say, in other words, that *balbuties* occurs for the most part from moisture, but rarely, from dryness. Not

---

[11]It is very clear, however, that in this passage Galen is using *ischnophonia* to refer strictly to the problem of thin voice, and not, like Aristotle, to stutering. Galen makes a strict distinction between voice and speech defects.

[12]In these passages, on sweating fever and dysentery, Hippocrates describes the tongue as *hypotraulos,* which is literally rendered into Latin as *subbalbus* (somewhat *balbus*). Dr. Wright, evidently taking this for *subalbus,* mistranslated "whitish."

[13]The examples given by Mercurialis in his Ch. 6 ("they say *pretium* for *precium*") show that he is referring to the substitution of palatalized t for the affricated stop č; and of l for a strongly trilled r.

only is this just what Avicenna seems to state expressly, but Aristotle certainly said the same, *On the History of Animals iv.9,* where he wrote that *balbutiēs* occurs most often in children, on account of the moisture and laxity of their tongues.

[Instrumental causes:] Moreover *balbutiēs* occurs when the tongue is either longer than it ought to be, as Galen said, *Aphorisms vi.32*[14] (although this rarely happens); or when it turns out too thick and too swollen; or when teeth are either missing, or arranged in bad order; or when the lips have been mutilated; or when the nostrils or windpipe are obstructed by a swelling of inflammation.

Chief among the external causes of defective speech is cold air. Indeed Aristotle, *Problems xi,* said that cold impedes speech by three causes. Firstly, because that which is cold, condenses. Secondly, because cold dulls the native heat, and consequently the motor faculty. And thirdly, because it ties the tongue, as it were; for the same author, *On the Parts of Animals ii.17,* said that for the act of speech to be carried through, it is highly necessary for the tongue to be made free and unimpeded. Thus a cold climate can prevent whole peoples from speaking correctly. It happens in this way that the speech in certain localities may be corrupted by a certain as it were hereditary affection in the people.[15]

Beyond other affections, those of the mind are apt to induce *balbutiēs*. It has been found out through experience, and both Galen and Aristotle have confirmed as well, that it may be induced by fear and similarly by anger, for one is accustomed to see many people who, while growing warm at the onset of excessive rage, sometimes become *balbi,* as indeed they are also driven to mutter under their breath. Deep thought can do the same, as also too much wakefulness, immoderate Venus; all of which, since they strongly injure the brain and all the nerves, bring on in consequence a detriment of speech.

Incessant drunkenness, however, impedes speech most of all, as Aristotle, *Problems iii,* and Galen, *Aphorisms vi.32,* have very clearly shown. There are even foods which by a certain property seem to obstruct the speech of children, for Raby Moses[16] writes, *Aphorisms part xx,* that children must be kept away from eating nuts, because they corrupt their speech.

For the rest, there is no need of signs by which to recognize defects of speech; but to become thoroughly acquainted with the causes, it is necessary to bring both signs and great industry to bear. For those who are silenced from birth on account of deafness are recognized, both by the fact that they are unmoved by noise or sound, and also that they have no defect in either the tongue or the mouth.

---

[14]Galen actually said "shorter."

[15]Cf. an interesting passage in Jean Bodin, *Method for the Easy Comprehension of History* (1566), trans. B. Reynolds (New York: Columbia U. P., 1945), Ch. 9, p. 343.

[16]I.e., Rabbi Moses Maimonides.

Although Aristotle, *Problems xi.2,* writes that mutes speak (or emit a noise) from their nostrils, because they are repressed in the mouth; [and that] they are surely repressed in the mouth because the tongue is of no use to them.

Those, however, who become mute either by the infliction of a wound, or on account of a slackening of the muscles of the tongue, are recognized by the very diseases which occurred prior to that: namely, by an apoplexy, or some antecedent illness of the kind.

Moreover those who can hardly speak, and are called *mogilaloi* by the Greeks, are recognized because, if the tongue is inspected, that bridle, commonly called the *philetum,* is particularly awkward and inept. For as delivered in Meletius, *On the Nature of Men,* since it was necessary for the tongue to form out the letters by its unhampered motion toward this or that part, nature decreed that it be allowed to do this freely; but lest it be too loose, and swing to and fro, she tied it to the mouth by a certain bridle, which prevents it from slipping.[17] But if a bridle of this kind is longer than it should be, so as to bind the tongue down too tightly, the latter is impeded in its ability to carry out the motions against the palate necessary for the proper articulation of the voice. Where this bridle is in fact too small it is recognized, because when the tongue is raised, it seems tied to nothing; just as, conversely, if the bridle is too great it is recognized, because it clasps much of the tongue, and will tightly hold it back from moving.

Hesitancy of the tongue, or *ischnophonia,*[18] whenever it occurs from diminished heat of that part, is recognized most evidently from this: that whenever they speak quietly and with delay, the impediment always appears greater. In fact, when they speak with a raised voice, and forcefully, then they deliver more unimpeded speech; because out of this motion and great voice, the muscles which move the tongue grow warm, and are therefore more easily moved.[19]

If the *balbutiēs* occurs from abundant moisture of the parts, such people are recognized because they are sleepy, dull of wit, have almost no memory, and always emit a great quantity of saliva while speaking.

If speech has been weakened either on account of the loss of teeth, or mutilation of the lips, or some disease of the nose, this is easily recognized by its own signs.

Mutes who are at the same time deaf are never cured; and therefore one of the miracles which our Savior performed was when he cured that deaf-mute in Matthew 15. But if muteness or loss of speech arises from too great laxity of the muscles because of abundant moisture, a problem of this kind is cured not only by the labors of a physician, but also at times spontaneously by nature. For it has been related that Maximilian, son of the Emperor Frederick III, was entirely speechless

---

[17]Cf. Galen, *On the Usefulness of the Parts of the Body,* trans. M. T. May (Ithaca: Cornell U. P., 1968), p. 523.

[18]A specific reference to stuttering.

[19]Although not noted in the text, this is from Aristotle, *Problems xi.35.*

and mute up to the ninth year of his age, but nevertheless acquired, by benefice of nature, not only speech, but indeed great eloquence; certainly it must be judged that in his case the fault traced its origin to abundant moisture, which by the advance of age, was consumed. So when we read that various people, although mute, suddenly acquired speech on account of either fear or anger, it must not be thought that this was accomplished by any chance or miracle, but in this way: that the impediment caused by moisture was removed.

Thus a natural *balbuties* of speech, whichever kind it be, is difficult to cure, just as that which occurs by some adventitious disease is not so difficult of cure. But what I said about a loss of speech which can be cured spontaneously by nature, must also be considered to apply to *balbuties*.

.

.

.

On this point, before I enter upon the cure, three problems occur. The first of which is, why was it said by Hippocrates, *Aphorisms vi.32,* that *balbi* are subject to diarrhea? Second, why did Hippocrates, *2 Epidemics 5 and 6,* also say that *balbi* are good?[20] (For Aristotle also writes in his *Physiognomy* that a heavy and delayed speech is the sign of a moderate mind.) Third, why in the same passages did Hippocrates say that *balbi* are subject to melancholy? (Something which has been confirmed by Avicenna, *iii fen 1.4.18,* as well.) For it seems almost beyond reason, that those with a brain of great moisture (of which type are *balbi*) can suffer from melancholy, which is a dry humor.

To the first it must be answered, in no other way than as Galen interpreted it in his commentary to that aphorism, that *balbi* of course necessarily have either a moist brain or a moist tongue. If they are of moist brain, the pituitous excrements which have precipitated from the head into the stomach, and consequently into the intestines, cause diarrhea, something which is delivered as tradition by Hippocrates in his book *On the Internal Affections.* Further, Avicenna surely said, *i fen 4.5.5,* that *balbi* often suffer a choleric passion for this reason as well. Moreover, if such people are *balbi* from excessive moisture of the tongue, they necessarily have a moist stomach, since the tongue shares a common skin with the stomach. And an affection certainly familiar to the stomach, as Galen says, is diarrhea.

To the second it must be replied that *balbi* are good on this account: because those who are of crooked character are so because of their hot and dry spirits. Since, on account of these, the mind is moved quickly, it does not give proper attention to things; whence also they lack prudence, and are consequently of bad

---

[20]The passages referred to are very obscure. The word "good" has sometimes been taken in the sense of "safe" (from the epidemic).

character. From this it happens that they are most sly and crooked in hot and dry regions, where huge beasts and wild animals are also born. Where the spirits are moist, however, the contrary happens, because since such people cannot be moved quickly, and since they pay greater attention, and do not have those quick motions, it happens, as is only fitting, that they are of moderate minds and correct character.

Most difficult of all, however, is the third and last problem: that is, why was it said by Hippocrates that *balbi* are melancholic, and suffer from melancholy diseases? Moreover the matter is rendered more difficult by the authority of Galen, *Aphorisms vii.40,* who, expounding that opinion of Hippocrates (in which the latter writes that if someone suddenly becomes incontinent of tongue,[21] he is melancholic), says that he knows not how incontinence of tongue might indicate a melancholic; and nevertheless adds below, almost as if taking refuge in the properties of things, that perhaps this is because, just as a quartan paroxysm occurs from a melancholy humor, so also from melancholy occurs incontinence of tongue. Since Jerome Cardan[22] also saw that this opinion was difficult, he said with a certain vanity of his own, that "incontinence of tongue" in Hippocrates must be interpreted as insolent and abusive speech; as if those who are insolent of speech, and say obscene things, were melancholics. But so far is Hippocrates from understanding anything of the kind by "incontinence of tongue," that if he had said it, he would have been no less vain than Cardan. For Aristotle, using almost the same words as Hippocrates, says that in children the tonge *becomes incontinent from moisture and weakness*.

Avicenna, *iii fen 1.4.18,* seems to have attributed the whole cause to heat of the heart, as if all *balbi,* who are of very moist brain, were also of very hot heart; and that therefore, since the heart is very hot, melancholy humors occur from the moisture upon which this heat continually acts[23]; and consequently, that when humors of this kind abound, melancholic illnesses arise at the same time. But neither can this opinion of Avicenna lighten the difficulty of the problem. First, because it has not been disclosed by any authority of the ancients that those of moist brain are of hot heart at the same time; nay, it would certainly seem that the case must be contrary, that a huge moisture of the brain would dull any heat of the body.[24a]

---

[21] Galen explains this expression (*akrates glossa* in Greek) as a very feeble, perhaps paralyzed tongue; it is used in the same way with respect to other parts of the body.

[22] In his commentaries to the *Aphorisms,* this one numbered vii.38; Hieronymus Cardanus, *Opera* (Lyon, 1663), v.8, p. 558.

[23] Avicenna's words are ". . . the heat of the heart becomes generative of black bile [melancholy] . . . and the moisture of the brain [becomes] susceptive of the impressions of that which is generated in the heart . . . ."

[24a] Avicenna merely says that *balbi,* among other types, are *predisposed* to this *(praeparati ad ipsum),* implying that melancholy will strike them *if* the heart should grow hot (e.g., in times of intense emotion).

But even if the statement that *balbi* are hot of heart be granted, it is not necessary that a melancholy humor occur, because there can also be an occurrence of yellow bile, as it has often been said that the bilious are hot of heart. For this reason it seems to me that Aristotle explained this better than anyone else in that passage, *Problems xi.38,* where, asking why the hesitant of tongue were melancholics, he wrote that all melancholics have quick motions of the imagination, and that *balbi*[24b] therefore, since they do have these quick motions, are melancholy as well. He says also, moreover, that *balbi* have quick motions because, since the instruments of the tongue itself are weak, and cannot exactly follow the concepts of the mind, it happens that the mind's motions always anticipate those of the tongue, and hence the impediment of tongue.

But neither can it be clearly gathered from these words of Aristotle why *balbi* really are subject to melancholy diseases, unless we should now also add that *balbi,* since they cannot speak as they desire, and as reason dictates, as if growing angry with themselves, and dreading to speak in the presence of others, are sad; and there is no doubt that this sadness and fear causes them a great production of melancholy, and subjects them in consequence to melancholic illnesses.

.

.

.

The treatment of defective speech is applied in children only when they have already been weaned, since before that time it cannot be known whether their speech is defective or not; and further, because it also often happens that children are *balbi* up until their sixth or seventh year, and are nonetheless spontaneously cured; on account of which, once it is certain that a spontaneous end is not to be put to the disease, treatment must be entered into immediately.

Those who are mute and deaf at the same time must be dismissed altogether. But if speech had been lost on account of a slackening of the tongue because of excessive moisture, the same cure must be applied, as in *balbutiēs.* And therefore when treating of the cure of *balbutiēs,* I shall be delivering that of muteness at the same time.

If the child be impeded in speech from an excessive attachment of the bridle, all efforts must be concentrated in a manual operation alone. Galen indeed writes that midwives used to cut away that membrane, called the bridle, with their nails[25];

[24b] Aristotle uses the word *ischnophonoi,* which in the *Problems* specifically means stutterers (see the definitions of terms in xi.30).

[25] On the widespread survival of this custom throughout Europe at the close of the 19th century, see Arthur Chervin, "Traditions Populaires relatives à la Parole," *Révue des Traditions Populaires, 15* (Mai 1900), pp. 241–263; also see I. M. Cullum, "An Old Wives' Tale," *British Medical Journal* (Sept. 19, 1959), pp. 497–498.

but whether on account of the unskillfulness of our own midwives, or whether it sometimes happens that this operation by itself is insufficient, it is necessary that another operation be applied. Cornelius Celsus, *vii.12,* a great expert in the art of surgery, puts forward a cure also proposed by Aëtius.[26] Moreover, it is an operation of this kind: elevate the tongue toward the palate, so that it touches it; thence stretch the membrane with a very light hook; afterwards cut all the way through with a very sharp knife, in such fashion, nevertheless, that the veins are in no way injured. This done, the mouth is to be rinsed out with posca[27]; next, powder of frankincense must be sprinkled on, and manna.[28] Thereafter the wound must be cared for, if necessary, like other wounds.

Cornelius Celsus adds one thing more: that speech is restored, for the most part, as soon as this membrane has been cut away; but sometimes, nevertheless, it is not, because although what should be done is constant, yet what comes to pass is not.

For the rest, in practice, there is often fear of profuse bleeding from the injury of a vein in making the incision. If this is feared, Avicenna advises, and most prudently, that the membrane itself not be cut, but perforated toward the root with a needle, and that a thread be drawn down by this needle, and tied. For this thread, if tightened daily, amputates the membrane gently, and in a short time. And this is a most agreeable method. When the membrane has actually been severed its remains are consumed with either Egyptian ointment or drying powders, lest it coalesce again.

In the treatment of each case of *balbutiēs,* however, there must be diligent inspection to determine exactly what the chief cause is. Because if a polyp of the nose is causing it, all attention ought to be directed toward treatment of the latter. If it should occur from mutilation of the lips, no hope remains. If from a tooth having been knocked out, there is this one way only: an ivory tooth should be prepared, and put in place of the missing one, and secured to the remaining teeth; after the tooth grows back, [the ivory one] is removed. This remedy is of great service to both children and men.

If this defect has been caused by a fault of the brain, or the tongue, or the muscles, the defect arises either from dryness, or from excessive moisture and cold. If from dryness, as happens in fevers and after frenzies, care must be taken that both the tongue and the beginning of the spinal marrow be moistened by every means. To moisten the tongue a gargling of woman's milk is useful; it is also often useful to dampen the tongue with water of mallows, to which oil of sweet almonds should be admixed, and if leaves of water-lily *(nimphaea)* are boiled together in

---

[26]*Tetrabiblos,* Bk. II, Serm. iv, Ch. 36.

[27] A mixture of vinegar and water.

[28] Manna: vegetable juice hardened into grains. Cf. Pliny, *Natural History xxix.6.38.,* par. 119.

water, the greatest aid will be afforded. Liniments which can soothe the spine or beginning of the spinal marrow are good:

℞: of pork lard, mallow soaked in

    water, chicken fat .... each 1 ounce.

    of oil of sweet almonds, of water-lily .... each ½ ounce.

    of saffron .... ½ scruple.

Mix in the mortar and let a liniment be made.[29]

Much greater zeal must be applied when *balbutiēs* occurs from the moisture and cold of the tongue, both because this defect occurs more frequently, and because there is need of many aids to combat it; and what I shall say as to its cure must equally be applied to those who become mute from a slackening brought on by excessive moisture. The chief aim in this treatment is to heat and dry out the tongue, brain, and muscles which move the tongue. Since the tongue and its muscles can in fact be dried out mainly by dissipating the moisture with which they are saturated, or by diverting the latter into other parts of the body, therefore attention will have to be paid to all of these, in order to dry out the moistures completely. For the thorough accomplishment of this, aids are surely to be sought from dietetics, pharmaceutics, and surgery.[30]

First, therefore, once the treatment has been undertaken, it must be seen to that the patient remain in air which is warm and dry; and it is perhaps on this account that when that *balbus* in Herodotus consulted the oracle, how he might cure his *balbutiēs,* it was answered him that he go to Lybia, a region very hot and very dry.

There must be more waking than sleeping.

Concerning the passions of the mind, it is clear that anger is to be avoided, because, as I said, it is reported that many have lapsed into *balbutiēs* through anger alone. For the rest, concerning fear, it is a very pretty question whether the physician treating *balbutiēs* must love fear, or shun it; for on the one hand there is reason for it to be shunned entirely, since there is no doubt that fear freezes; it is for this reason, I said earlier, that those in fear are *balbi.* But on the other hand examples are given in the historians in which children and also even men, who had

---

[29]Recipes of this type evidently go back a long way. Nicolus Falcutius Florentinus, in his *Sermo Tertius de Membris Capitis* (Venice, 1490), tract. viii cap. 21, quotes the following from "Haly" (i.e., Ali ibn al Abbas, Persian physician, d. 994): "When it is from dryness it is cured with a gargarism of the milk of a woman who has a daughter, and with oil of violets or almonds, or of cucumbers, and the spondyles (vertebra) of the neck are emplastered. You shall employ humectations, either of chicken fat, or fat of a sheep's tail, or of unsalted pork lard. And you shall have mixed these fats with oil of violets or water-lilies, and violet and water-lily flowers mixed by halves with froth of (citrons?).

[30]From here to the end, Mercurialis conceives his treatments according to the "six non-naturals" mentioned briefly in our introduction (see p. 3). They are taken up in the following order: air, sleep, passions of mind and body, exercise, excretions, food, and drink.

earlier been mute, were said to have acquired speech. For Pausanias tells us that a certain Batus, a mute, having spied a lion in the desert, was struck with the greatest fear, and immediately procured speech.[31] It is also related that Athis, son of Croesus, fearing that his father was to be killed by Cyrus, acquired speech as soon as he realized the danger. Therefore, since these things seem to have happened in the course of nature, and not by miracle, it also seems that muteness or *balbutiēs* may sometimes be cured by terror excited by the physician.

It seems to me that the problem (not heretofore proposed) must be solved in this way: that fear is of two kinds, the one named *agonia* by the Greeks, by us *trepidation*; the other certainly that which by us is properly called *fear*, and *phobos* by the Greeks.

Trepidation is the fear of men about to set out upon some great matter, which kind of fear is more often called by the name *timor*. In trepidation, as delivered in Aristotle, *Problems xi.53,* there is as it were a certain kind of shame *(pudor)*. Hence, just as in shame the parts around the breast grow exceedingly warm, as indicated by their redness, so thus, says he, it is fitting that those in trepidation are beset about the breast and face with heat, on account of which the voice grows deep.

With those in fear proper, however, it is otherwise, since the parts of the breast and the upper parts grow cold; the heat moreover seeks the lower parts. Whence Aristotle, *Problems vii.4,*[32] said that in those in fear, the semen, urine, and faeces flow of their own accord, because the heat forced down to the lower parts excites those excretions.

With this solution proposed, therefore, it is easy to untie the knot: namely, that simple fear not only is no help for *balbutiēs,* but rather augments it, because it freezes the tongue, breast, and upper parts, as is recognized from their pallor. Trepidation, on the other hand, can be of the greatest help in both *balbutiēs* and muteness, because with the breast and upper parts heated, it is not to be doubted that the excessive moisture can be lifted, and along with it the weakness which arises from poverty of native heat, whence it can be generally useful to induce this trepidation in children.

The body must be exercised as much as possible; certainly the voice must be exercised in particular; and if there is anything which may benefit *balbi* and stutterers,[33] it is a continuous loud and clear speaking.[34] Of this, example is given

---

[31]This is generally considered to be the same Battus as mentioned in Herodotus. (See footnote 1, above.) Cf. also Jacob Grimm, *Teutonic Mythology,* 4 ed. (London, 1880), ch. xv. 5, v. I, p. 388.

[32]Cf. also xxvii. 1, 3, and 10.

[33]*Haesitantibus:* another specific reference to stutterers.

[34]On vociferation as an aid to health, see Galen, *De Sanitate Tuenda i.11, v.10, ii.2, iii.2*; in *Galen's Hygiene,* trans. R. M. Green (Springfield, Ill.: Charles C. Thomas, 1951), pp. 54, 54–55, 87, 103–105, 219–220.

of the great Demosthenes, who, as Plutarch tells us in his biography, and in the booklet *Of Ten Orators,* conquered his *balbutiēs* by exercise of the voice alone and by formal oratory. For he gave 10,000 drachmas to Neoptolemus the actor, who taught him how to recite many lines in one breath: namely, that he should continually recite verses while climbing and running, with pebbles in his mouth.[34a]

Venus must be abstained from, if they are men; children however are to abstain from the use of baths; whence mothers who are accustomed to often wash the head for their *balbi* children do badly, since they are increasing the moisture and the cause of this defect. Care must be taken that the bowels flow daily, if not by nature then at least by art.

Wine must be abstained from, or it must be used weak and in small quantity. For food they are to use aromatic, salty, and sharp edibles, abstaining from the use of pastries, nuts, and fish; and, in a word, the entire principle of life must be to dry out and to warm. When this principle of life has been established, the child should be purged.

To begin with, if the bowels have not flowed spontaneously, the following little potion should be dissolved:

R̥:   of sage leaves, of betony .... each ½ minim.
      of coriander .... 1 dram.
      of senna leaves .... 2 scruples.

Let a decoction be made according to the direction, then

R̥:   of the said decoction .... 2½ ounces.
      of laxative honey of roses .... 2 or 2½ ounces.

Mix; let a potion be made. Then the body should be prepared for purging:

R̥:   of sage leaves, of oregano, of stachys .... each ½ minim.

Let a decoction be made according to the direction, then

R̥:   of the said decoction .... 3 ounces.
      of plain oxymel[35] .... 2 ounces.
      of syrup of betony, of stachys .... each ½ ounce.

Mix; let a potion be made. After the body has been prepared, it should be purged, and in this purging, if it is suitable to use pills, they should be preferred to other medicaments.

R̥:   of pills of hiera[36] with agaric .... 1½ scruples.
      of pills of cochee[37] .... 1 scruple.

Mix; let pills be made to the number of five.

[34a] See H. Holst, "Demosthenes' Speech Impediment," *Symbolae Osloenses*, fasc. 4 (1926), 11–25.

[35] A mixture of vinegar and honey.

[36] A strong purgative.

[37] A very strong purge for the head.

That these may be swallowed the more easily by children, they may be hidden in a little cake, or some jam; but if they have refused the pills, the following potion must be given:

R̥: of agaric done into tablets .... 2 scruples.

of cloves .... 4 grains.

Let them be infused in water of stachys or betony; then, having been pressed out, add three drams of diacatholicon,[38] one ounce of laxative honey of roses with a cordial decoction. Let a potion be made.

When the body has been purged, care should be taken that those parts along with the brain be dried out still further; and for this, medicaments which are drawn into the nostrils, and sneezings, are beneficial.

R̥: of beetroot juice .... ½ ounce.

of betony juice .... 1 ounce.

of water of corianders .... ½ pound.

Let them be mixed and drawn into the nostrils.

When the child's body has been purged for a little while, care should be taken that the head and the tongue be continually dried out. The head is continually dried out by a cautery applied to the nucha[39]; a more effective remedy than this is hardly found in this category. Similarly, for drying out the head, vesicatories[40] applied behind the ears, and kept there for a long period, are most effective. For drying out the tongue, it is of advantage to rub it sometimes with honey, sometimes with salt, and most often with sage.[41] Usage attests how very effective this is for doing away with *balbutiēs*.

And let this be the end of those affections which pertain to the motor faculty.

---

[38] An all-purpose purgative composed of several ingredients.

[39] (From an Arabic word): the beginning of the spinal marrow.

[40] Blistering agents.

[41] Dr. Wright read "saliva" for "salvia."

THE

SEATS and CAUSES

OF

DISEASES

INVESTIGATED BY ANATOMY;

IN FIVE BOOKS,

CONTAINING

A Great Variety of DISSECTIONS, with REMARKS.

TO WHICH ARE ADDED

Very ACCURATE and COPIOUS INDEXES of the
PRINCIPAL THINGS and NAMES therein contained.

TRANSLATED from the LATIN of

JOHN BAPTIST MORGAGNI,

Chief Profeſſor of Anatomy, and Preſident of the Univerſity at PADUA,

By BENJAMIN ALEXANDER, M.D.

IN THREE VOLUMES.

VOL. I.

LONDON,

Printed for A. MILLAR; and T. CADELL, his Succeſſor, in the Strand;
and JOHNSON and PAYNE, in Pater-noſter Row.

MDCCLXIX.

diforder ; to wit, that his diforder was accuftom'd to be remov'd, if any body breath'd into his ear.   But it muft, at leaft, have been a very different affection ; nor would our patient have fent for three phyficians to attend him, if he could have been cur'd by fo eafy a remedy.

38. I muft alfo add fomething upon ftammering.   For in the twenty-firft obfervation our Sanctorius is quoted as faying thefe things (y) : " That there " are, in the middle region of the palate, that is, in the fourth bone of the " upper jaw, in all whom he had feen to that time, who could not exprefs " the letter R, two foramina, which are by no means found open and ob- " vious in thofe who are under the influence of this difeafe ; therefore, that " the immediate caufe, which fuppofes others granted, will be thofe two " paffages being open."   Nay, truly, not being open, any one would fay, who fhould read this paffage with any tolerable care, and at the fame time attend to the argument prefix'd to the obfervation, which is this, " That " ftammering depends, fometimes, on the defect of the foramina of the " fourth bone of the upper jaw."   But if he fhould examine the paffage, in Sanctorius himfelf, he would find that he has written the very contrary to thefe things : for he fays, that he had feen, in perfons who ftammer'd, thofe two foramina, " which are by no means found fo open and obvious in thofe " who are free from this diforder ; wherefore, the immediate caufe, which " fuppofes others granted, will be," fays he, " thefe two meatus, or foramina, " more open than they ought to be."   See, I befeech you, with what care- leffnefs the words of authors are fometimes copied : yet this is the paffage of the Sepulchretum, with a view to which very excellent men have written, " That Sanctorius had attributed ftammering to the defect of the ductus in- " cifivus, in the Sepulchretum of Bonetus, I. p. 473."   But if they had chofen rather to look into the chapter of Sanctorius, which is quoted in the fame place (z), without doubt, they would neither have believ'd that, nor would have underftood the ductus incifivus.   For Sanctorius, a little below, adds thefe words : " As I faid that in the middle region of the palate, two fora- " mina were obferv'd, which are the caufes of ftammering, fo, in like man- " ner, I obferve larger foramina, near the teeth, (yet in all thefe perfons, " congenial with their original formation) through which a pituita diftilling " and moiftening the tongue, on its anterior part, makes an impediment in " the fpeech, from whence they become lifping and fhort-tongu'd ;" fo evi- dent is it, that from the meatus being very open behind the dentes incifores, he had accounted for the habit of lifping only, and not that of ftammering, of which the queftion is in this obfervation : and how thefe two kinds of im- pediment to the fpeech differ one from another, the learned fcholia to the next and twenty-fourth obfervation, will fhew.

You will afk here, why this fecond obfervation of Sanctorius is omitted in the Sepulchretum, whereas the firft is given there, though erroneoufly ? And in like manner, what can thefe two foramina be then, in that fame fourth bone, and in the middle region of the palate, which are more open in perfons who ftammer than in others ?   And at length, how much regard

(y) Sect. 22.   (z) Meth. vitand. error. l. 3. c. 9.

is to be paid to thefe obfervations of Sanctorius ?   I do not doubt but it was owing to the fame carelefnefs which perverted the firft, that the fecond was omitted.

And as to the foramina in that middle region of the palate, I do not remember to have feen any thing of them in the many dry and prepar'd heads that I have examin'd; nor do I at this prefent time fee any fuch thing in any of thefe heads which I have before me now, while I write; nor yet fhould I eafily believe, that in fo great a number of heads, as have come into my hands, I never happen'd to light on one that had belong'd to a ftammerer, in which, doubtlefs, I fhould have feen thefe foramina very plainly, inafmuch as they were very open, and obvious in them, though in others very obfcure.

But although it is natural to fufpect, that what Sanctorius had by chance obferv'd, in fome ftammerers, he had transferr'd to all; and although difficulties are not wanting to prevent our affenting thereto, from reading his words, and even from the very things that he fays, in confirmation of what he advances; for he confeffes, that even they in whom the mouth naturally and conftantly overflows with pituita, are not, for that reafon, ftammerers, nor lifpers; yet on account of his well-known excellence in other matters, it will be more juft and fair, I think, not to pronounce any thing abfolutely on the point, before the queftion fhall have been accurately canvafs'd by fkilful anatomifts, who have examin'd the heads of many ftammerers and lifpers to this purpofe.

So the celebrated Delius (a), having found a double uvula in a certain perfon, who had been a ftammerer, very prudently admonifh'd anatomifts, that they fhould enquire, whether other perfons who ftammer have any fault or diforder about the uvula, or tonfils.   And if this were done, I conjecture, being induc'd thereto by very probable arguments, it would be found, that even in him who was a ftammerer, the impediment could not, juftly, have been imputed to the double uvula.   For there are many examples extant of this duplication, which you know I have pointed out, on a former occafion (b); nor Zerbus; nor thofe whom Slevogtius commends; nor I myfelf, at leaft in that perfon whom I diffected at Bologna, have heard any thing of an impediment of this kind, in the fpeech, notwithftanding almoft all of us enquir'd diligently what inconveniences had attended this duplication of the uvula: and without doubt that Lucretia of Zerbus, if fhe had pronounc'd vitioufly in this way, would never have given herfelf up to the art of finging, nor would have " delighted very much," in the practice, as he himfelf teftifies that fhe did.

But it is a very fuppofable cafe, that ftammering may fometimes arife from confiderable defects about the os hyoides: and indeed I find the very learned Hahnius has advanc'd this doctrine (c); that from the figure of this bone being deprav'd, " perfons become ftammerers, lifpers, and dumb." Nor indeed does it feem poffible, that the directions of the mufcles which move the tongue can be chang'd, without making the motions of the tongue,

<hr/>

(a) Act. N. C. Tom. 8. obf. 106.   (c) Commerc. Litter. A. 1736. Hebd. 31.
(b) Epift. Anat. 10. n. 21.   n. 1. ad § 25.

in

in fome meafure, deviate from the law of nature.   And if Kerckringius (d) had written what was true, concerning the os hyoides, when he fays, " that " in fœtuffes, not fo much as a cartilage of it appears;" I fhould not have doubted, but it was for this reafon, that little children begin to fpeak very late after their birth; and when they have begun, " attempt only half-words," or " fpeak their words ftammeringly," as Minucius Felix (e), and Albius Tibullus (f), have faid, in order to exprefs their manner of fpeaking.   But the illuftrious Albinus (g) fufficiently fhews, how late this bone, which is the fulcrum of the tongue, and fome of its mufcles, becomes perfectly compleat on all fides, and entirely bony.

And to our Molinetti it feem'd (h), " that the infant did not fpeak imme- " diately after it was born," for this reafon, becaufe the ftyliform procefs, from which the ftylogloffus, and ftylohyoideus mufcles, take their origin, " does not appear in a fœtus." Which if you underftand, fo as to believe, that he denied the exiftence of this procefs in a fœtus; he certainly has blunder'd, as Caffebohmius teftifies (i), that he had feen it in a fœtus of four months, and Kerckringius (k) even in a fœtus of three months.   But if you fo underftand it, that by reafon of the flendernefs and flexibility of the cartilage, he did not confider it of any greater advantage in its prefent condition, particularly in order to fix fteadily, the origin and action of the mufcles, than if there had been none at all; you may by this means fufficiently protect his affertion, from what I faw, when I read over this letter again, would be objected to his opinion, taken from a very fingular obfervation of that moft excellent author Haller (l).   For he, in a man who was about fifty years of age, and who had never labour'd under the leaft impediment in his fpeech, found the ftyliform procefs of the length of an inch and half, being bony in the lower half of it, and in the upper part of it cartilaginous.   But you, to omit this fuppofition, that in the man whom Haller obferv'd, the mufcles we fpeak of might poffibly have their origin, in part, from the neighbouring temple bone, as both Valfalva (m) and I (n) have fometimes found its fellow, the ftylopharyngæus, taking its origin; you certainly underftand, that the cartilage, which according to the increafe of years, was fo much thicker and ftronger, ought not to be compar'd with that which Molinetti, in confequence of its being fo flender and foft, confider'd as none at all, in new-born infants: and you know, at the fame time, to what, and to how many mufcles, fome of the cartilages of the larynx give origin.   But in regard to this defence of Molinetti, you yourfelf will determine.

I indeed think, that from what caufes foever the ftammering of little children is to be accounted for, it may be imputed to many more caufes, than thofe which are made mention of; and I believe that from the fame caufes, the ftammering of adults arifes, as often as ever it happens, that the increafing age cannot overcome one, or more, of thefe caufes.   And it will certainly

(d) Ofteogen. c. 11.
(e) in Octavio.
(f) l. 2. Eleg. 5. v. 94.
(g) Icon. Off. Fœt. ad Fig. 152.
(b) Differt. Anat. Pathol. l. 2. c. 1.
(i) De Aure Hum. tr. 1. § 43.

(k) Ofteogen. c. 5.
(l) in Differt. Willigii infcript. obf. Botan. &c. § 2.
(m) Vid. Epift. Anat. 11. n. 4.
(n) Ibid. n. 8.

be of advantage to enquire into these causes, in young children, since, from the universal stammering among them, it will be more easy to observe the causes of it, so that we may endeavour to distinguish them more sagaciously, in adults, and, as far as it can be done, sometimes, to diminish, or remove them.

39. Lastly, as to what relates to the twenty-third section, which is on the angina, it is very surprising, that no observation is produc'd in this whole section, of that most violent and frequent disorder of the larynx, and the neighbouring fauces, from which it may appear, what has been found in those who have died of a true angina.   For some of those observations that are produc'd relate to the lungs, or to these, and the gland thymus, being stuff'd up with blood; the first of which, by their weight, drew the aspera arteria downwards, and the latter, by its encreas'd bulk, compress'd it; others relate to the disorders of the brain, or of other parts; so that any person, who was unexperienc'd, might suspect, whether this disorder ever belongs to the larynx and fauces.   But certainly in the angina, an external tumour often about the fauces, or an internal tumour, as I have more than once seen, and have order'd to be cautiously incis'd, as it already contain'd pus, and in the larynx also, that which was the first cause of performing the operation of laryngotomy, as it is call'd, are sufficient proofs of an angina existing, from an inflammation, which occupies those parts above mention'd; and indeed, to pass over the muscles, by which the arytenoid cartilages are brought close to each other, unless you can suppose, that the glands, which moisten the larynx, are entirely free from those disorders, which happen to other glands of the same kind; it will plainly appear that it cannot be otherwise, but that inflammations, sometimes, and those of the most dangerous kind, seize upon our arytenoid glands, for instance, by the swelling of which the air-passage, that is there naturally narrow, must be shut up, or of course much obstructed.

However, I do not say this, because I believe that you think otherwise; but for this reason only, that you may understand this to be one of those disorders, the seats of which are peculiar, and sometimes more, sometimes less, dangerous in their nature and effects; and though every one of these circumstances ought to be enquir'd into with earnestness, and care, yet that they do not seem to be enquir'd into by dissection, so much as the seats, causes, nature, and effects of other disorders are (o).   And this has not been done by me for this reason, because I once had not time to dissect a person who died of the true angina; and ever since that, I have not had it in my power, for want of subjects who died of the disorder (p): but with the spurious, perhaps, who certainly, however, did not die from this cause, I dissected one or two.   What I observ'd in the fauces and larynx of these patients, you will read over again in the fourth letter I sent you (q); and you may, in some measure, refer to the true angina, those things of which I made mention when I wrote on the hydrophobia (r).   Farewel.

(o) Vid. tamen Epist. 63. n. 16. & seq.   (q) n. 24. & seqq.
(p) Sed vid. Epist. 44. n. 3.   (r) Epist. 8. n. 19. & seqq.

Andrew Combe's Review of
M. Felix Viosin's book, *Causes and Cures of Stammering,*
from the *Phrenological Journal,*
1826, Vol. 4, No. 25, Edinburgh

Du Begaiement, ses Causes, &c., et Moyens Therapeutiques pour Prevenir, Modifier, ou Guerir cette Infirmité; par M. Felix Voisin, D. M. P.—*Paris, pp. 47.*

Stammering has generally been ascribed to some physical impediment in the tongue, the palate, or some other of the organs of speech; but it is easy to show that its cause is of a very different origin, and that it rarely, if ever, arises from simple malformation of the vocal organs.

It is justly observed by the author before us, who is (or was) himself afflicted to a great degree with this defect of speech, and who is therefore no very incompetent judge, that the anatomical inspection of the vocal organs does not demonstrate any vice of conformation. "The persons," says he,

> that I have seen, and who, like myself, spoke with difficulty, had not, as is alleged, the tongue larger than other people, nor its ligaments laxer, nor its frenum excessively long, nor the teeth so placed as to present any obstacle. It is incontestable, indeed, that all these lesions exist, and I have myself seen every one of them; but when they do exist, they give rise to phenomena totally different. To be convinced of this it is only necessary to examine the individuals in whom they present themselves. We shall remark, it is true, a greater or less alteration of pronunciation, but *never the characteristic symptoms of stammering.*

If physical malformation were really the general cause of stammering, the effect would necessarily be permanent, and would affect the same sounds every time they recurred; but the reverse of this is the truth; for it is well known that, on occasions of excitement, the stammerer often displays a fluency and facility of utterance the very opposite of his habitual state, and that, as Dr Voisin expresses it, *"lorsqu'ils "se mettent en colère, ils blasphement avec une énergie qui n'a point échappé aux hommes les moins observateurs."* P. 4. But passion or excitement can never remove a physical cause, make a large tongue small, set crooked teeth straight, or tighten the ligaments of the tongue, and then let these imperfections return as soon as the storm is over. Such causes, then, may make a person speak thick or low, or indistinctly, but his utterance will still be as equable and free from stammer as before, and therefore the true stammer must depend on a totally different antecedent.

Dr Voisin proves very clearly, that the real cause is irregularity in the nervous action of the parts which combine to produce speech. This is shown by analyzing speech. The natural sounds, or vowels, are simple, and require only one kind of muscular action for their production, hence they are almost always under command. The artificial, or compound sounds (hence denominated *con-sonants*) are complex, and require *several* distinct and successive combinations of a variety of muscles; and it is they alone that excite stammering. But it is *the brain* that directs and combines all voluntary notions, and consequently every disturbing cause, not local and not permanent, can affect the voluntary motions of speech only *through the medium of* the brain; and irregular action of the brain must thus be the indispensable antecedent or cause of the effect—stammering. This will be obvious on reviewing the *exciting* causes of that infirmity.

First, It is no unusual thing to see a person, who is perfectly fluent in conversation, and who has never been known to stammer, become grievously affected with it, if called upon unexpectedly to address a public audience. Every one will admit that, in this case, there is no physical impediment to utterance, but that the cause is in the brain, or organ of the mind, and that it consists in an irregular nervous impulse sent to the organs of speech, and proceeding from a *conflict* between the *desire* to speak well, the *fear* of speaking ill, or perhaps a consciousness of a paucity or bad arrangement of the ideas which he is expected to communicate, or it may be a dearth of words in which to clothe them. In every instance the *essential* circumstance is a conflict or absence of co-operation among the active faculties, necessarily giving rise to a *plurality,* instead of to a *unity,* of nervous impulses, and consequently to a *plurality,* instead of to a unity, of simultaneous muscular combinations; and the irregular plurality of purposes and of actions thence resulting constitutes exactly what is called stammering.

A striking illustration of the truth of this view is the fact, that stammering, or irregularity of action, is an affection not peculiar to the muscles concerned in the production of speech, but is common to these, and to all the muscles under the power of the will. Wherever two or more diverging purposes of nearly equal power assail the mind, and prompt to opposite courses of action at the same time, there stammering appears, whether it be in the muscles of the vocal organs, or in those of the feet. We recollect a ludicrous example of this in a boy at a dancing-school ball in the Assembly Rooms. He was dancing very easily and gracefully, and with much inward tranquillity and satisfaction, when, on a sudden, on raising his head, his wonder was attracted and dazzled by the unusual splendour of the chandeliers, which he had not before noticed. His feet continued to move, but with evidently less unity of purpose than before, and after making a few unmeaning and rather eccentric movements, or *stammering with his feet* instead of with his tongue, he fell on his back on the floor, and awoke from his reverie.

Secondly, A person unexpectedly beset by danger *stammers* from head to foot, till his presence of mind gives him an *unity* of purpose, and decides what he is to do. In this instance, it is undeniably the simultaneous existence of opposite mental impulses that produces the effect. For the same reason the sudden recollection, during an animated discourse, of something forgotten, causes a temporary stammer and unsteadiness of attitude. In short, a multiplicity of impulses causes contrariety of action, and contrariety of action constitutes *stammering*.

The influence which the encephalon exercises over pronunciation," says Dr Voisin, "is equally established by the observations continually furnished by orators, advocates, and public speakers. If the intellectual operations are carried on with rapidity, if the ideas are clear, numerous, and well-connected, the pronunciation will be free, easy, and agreeable; if, on the contrary, the march of intellect is slow and difficult, and the ideas are confused and ill arranged, the elocution will partake of the internal trouble, and the orator, thus accidentally a stammerer, will soon have fatigued his audience by his repetitions and disagreeable articulations.

We have seen the same thing arise from a deficient supply of words to clothe the ideas that presented themselves; the contrariety arising in this instance from the ineffectual struggle of a small organ of Language to keep pace with the workings of larger organs of intellect.

Thirdly, The effects of wine and spirituous liquors prove the influence of the brain in the production and cure of stammering.

Look at that individual, who, without committing any excess, is moderately excited by a few glasses of wine; *lately* he was sad, silent, and spiritless; *now,* what a metamorphosis! he is gay, talkative, and witty; let him continue to drink, and go beyond the measure of his necessities, his head will become embarrassed, and the fumes of the wine trouble his intellectual functions. *The muscles, subjected to the guidance of a will without power, contract feebly, and the most confused and marked stammering succeeds* to the fluent pronunciation so lately observed, and which depended on the powerful action of the brain on the organs of speech.

Fourthly, From the earliest antiquity accidental stammering has been noticed by physicians as frequently the precursor of apoplexy and palsy, which could only happen from the preceding affection of the brain acting on the organs of speech.

Fifthly, M. Voisin himself remarks the well-known fact, that stammerers are generally very sensitive and easily irritable, and, at the same time, timid and retiring; thus affording the essential contrariety of emotions in its strongest degree. M. Voisin forcibly delineates this state, when he says,

I shall never forget that, in 1813, when I had finished my studies, and was entering on life, my troubled countenance (*ma contenance mal assurée,*) my embarrassment and monosyllabic answers, and the silence which fear and timidity almost always enforced upon me, gave to many people such an idea of my character, that I may dispense with quoting the epithet which they were pleased to bestow upon me.

Sixthly, Certain emotions, by exciting the brain, direct such a powerful nervous influx upon the organs of speech, that not only delivers the stammerer from his infirmity for a time, but has even sufficed to deliver the dumb from their bondage, and enabled them to speak. Esquirol gives a curious example of this fact. A dumb man had long endured contempt and bad usage from his wife; but, being one day more grossly maltreated than usual, he got into such a furious rage, that he regained the use of his tongue, and repaid with usury the execrations which his tender mate had so long lavished upon him. This shows how closely the brain influences speech.

Seventhly, Speech is the conductor of ideas, and is useless where none exist. Accordingly it is noticed, that idiots, although they hear well, and have a sound conformation of the organs of speech, and a power of emitting all the natural sounds, are either dumb, or speak very imperfectly.

Eighthly, Under the influence of contending emotions, as is well observed by M. Voisin, the tongue either moves without firmness, or remains altogether immoveable. This, he says, occurs most frequently when Cautiousness or fear, and Veneration or respect, are the opposing feelings. Stammering from this cause diminishes perceptibly, and sometimes even disappears, in proportion as the individual regains his presence of mind and masters his internal impression.

> The observations, he adds, which I have the sad privilege of making on myself every day confirm what is here advanced. I have often intercourse with men for whom I feel so much respect, that it is almost impossible for me to speak to them when I appear before them. But if the conversation, of which they at first furnish the whole, goes on and becomes animated, recovering soon from my first emotion, I shake off all little considerations, and, raising myself to their height, I discuss with them *without fear,* and without the slightest difficulty in my pronunciation.

This indicates the supreme influence of the nervous influx on the movements of the vocal muscles, and it is curiously supported and illustrated by a fact mentioned by M. Itard, of a boy of eleven, who was excessively at fault whenever he attempted to speak in the presence of persons looking at him, but in whom the stammering instantly disappeared as soon as, by shutting out the light, he ceased to be visible. This is explicable only on the theory of opposite mental emotions.

Ninthly, As the individual advances in age, and acquires consistency and unity of character, the infirmity becomes less and less marked, and even frequently disappears altogether. In the same way it is generally more marked in the morning than in the evening, because the brain has not then assumed its full complement of activity, nor been exposed to the numerous stimuli which beset it in the ordinary labours of the day.

A late writer seems to us to mistake the effect for the cause, when he says that stammerers, being deprived of the means of communication with their fellows, *become* reserved and timid in society, and of exquisite sensibility; for, according to the view we have been unfolding, the natural timidity and sensibility, instead of being the effect, are in fact the chief causes of the stammer or defect in pronunciation. And we think this confirmed by his own observation, that old age is generally a cure, and that

> old men, when interrogated on the causes of the amendment, generally attribute it to their having become less hasty, or *much more moderate* and *considerate,* and in a much less hurry to force out their ideas.[1]

The cerebral and mental cause of stammering explains the effects of education and the rational mode of cure.

Speech being the vehicle of ideas, and of no use but to convey them, it is obvious that one important condition in securing a distinct articulation is to have previously acquired distinct ideas. Idiots, having few ideas, never learn to speak. For the same reason, children ought not to be forced to speak in the way that is generally done. This ill-timed haste has the opposite effect, for the subjects of it speak later and with greater confusion; and the extreme attention that is paid to their every word, dispenses them from distinct articulation, and causes a bad pronunciation for their whole lives. This is remarked very often in children brought up in towns. They speak earlier, but much less distinctly, than those reared in the country. Learning by rote is held by Dr Voisin to be very pernicious, as it accustoms the child to negligent and unmeaning pronunciation in his repetition of the same words.

It is remarked, indeed, that those who are late of speaking never spaek so distinctly as the others; but here the effect is often mistaken for the cause, for the child is long of speaking only because his vocal organs are *naturally* embarrassed, and not because the latter are embarrassed from the want of speech. If the organs were not constitutionally impeded, why should any one child be longer of speaking than another? The child that stammers has quite as much use for speaking as any other, and in general he is stimulated to an infinitely greater degree to exert his power of speech. Parents become uneasy, and, by their ill-judged efforts at hastening, often cause the very defect they seek to avoid.

From this view it will appear that the cure of stammering is to be looked for in removing the exciting causes, and in bringing the vocal muscles into harmonious action by *determined* and patient exercise. The opposite emotions, so generally productive of stammering, may, espeically in early life, be gradually got rid of by a judicious moral treatment,—by directing the attention of the child to the existence of these emotions as causes—by inspiring him with friendly confidence,—by exciting him resolutely to shun any attempt at pronunciation when he feels himself unable to master it,—*by his exercising himself when alone and free from emotion, in talking and reading aloud and for a length of time, so as to habituate the muscles to simultaneous and systematic action;* and we may add, as a very effectual

---

[1]Dictionnaire de Médécine, tome iii. p. 344.

remedy, by *increasing the natural difficulty in such a way as to require a* STRONG UNDIVIDED MENTAL EFFORT *to accomplish the utterance of a sound,* and thereby add to the amount of nervous energy distributed to the organs of speech. The practice of Demosthenes is a most excellent example. He cured himself of inveterate stammering by filling his mouth with pebbles, and accustoming himself to recitations in that state. It required strong local action, and a *concentrated attention,* to emit a sound without choking himself, or allowing the pebbles to drop from his mouth; and this was precisely the natural remedy to apply to *opposite and contending emotions and divided attention.*

Demosthenes adopted the other most effectual part of the means of cure. He exercised himself *alone,* and *free from distracting emotions,* to such a degree that he constructed a subterraneous cabinet on purpose for perfect retirement, and sometimes passed two and three months without ever leaving it, having previously shaven one half of his head, that he might not be able to appear in public when the temptation should come upon him. And the perfect success which attended this plan is universally known. His voice passed from a weak, uncertain, and unmanageable, to a full, powerful, and even melodious tone, and became so remarkably flexible as to accommodate itself with ease to the very numerous and delicate inflections of the Greek tongue. But as a complete cure, or harmonious action of the vocal muscles, can be obtained only be the repetiton of the muscular action till a habit or *tendency to act* becomes established, it is evident that *perseverance* is an essential element in its accomplishment, and that without this the temporary amendment obtained at first by the excitement consequent upon a trial of any means very soon disappears, and leaves the infirmity altogether unmitigated.

M. Itard, whom we have already mentioned, recommends very strongly, where it can be done, to force children to speak in a foreign language by giving them a foreign governess or tutor; and the propriety of this advice is very palpable when we consider that it requires a more powerful and concentrated effort to speak and to pronounce a foreign than a native tongue, and that it is precisely a strong, undivided, and long-continued mental effort that is necessary to effect a cure.

M. Itard regards weakness in the muscles of the voice as the cause of stammering, and he has invented, and used with much success, a small forked instrument which he places under the tongue, in order to give them support. We approve highly of the practice, but think his explanation of its efficacy likely to lead to error. To us it appears to serve the same purpose that the pebbles did in the mouth of the Grecian orator, viz. to solicit such an amount of nervous stimulus to the parts, and such an effort of attention as shall absorb the mind, and prevent its unity of purpose being divided by contrary emotions. And the proofs that this is the true source of the muscular debility are, that for all purposes except speaking, the movements of the lips and tongue are as powerful and as perfect as in any other individual, and that old age, which increases real debility, and which, therefore, ought to increase stammering if it arose from this cause, almost invariably cures it.

We think it right to notice this mistake in principle, as, from M. Itard's well-merited reputation, his practice is likely to be followed; and as every man will modify it according to his own lights, many, viewing it as a mere mechanical support, might do so in a wrong way, and produce mischief instead of benefit, and then blame him for misleading them.

It is scarcely necessary to add, that debility, in which this, in common with many other forms of nervous disease, often originates in the young, must be obviated by a due supply of nourishing food, country air, regular exercise, and last, though not least, by cheerful society, kindness, and encouragement. The use of Phrenology in enabling a stammerer to understand his own case, or a parent to direct the treatment of his child under this infirmity, is so obvious, that we reckon it unnecessary to dwell on it. By rendering the nature and modes of action of the mental powers clear and familiar, it aids us in removing every morbid affection of which the origin lies in them.

Chapter VII (Stammering)
from *A System of Elocution. . .* , Philadelphia, 1841

ANDREW COMSTOCK, M.D.

STAMMERING is a functional derangement of the organs of speech, which renders them incapable, under certain circumstances, of promptly obeying the commands of the will.

In a majority of cases, the cause of this affection operates through the medium of the mind.

Stammering is cured by a regular course of hygienic elocution. But, as the disease exists under a variety of forms, it requires a variety of treatment. And, as the treatment is *medico-elocutional,* he who would apply it successfully, must unite the skill of the elocutionist with that of the *physician.* The idea that non-medical men are capable of discharging the duties of applying the remedies to complicated complaints of the human body, is a *sui generis* in logic, and a bane in the practice of the healing art.

As a *full* consideration of the subject of stammering is not compatible with the design of *this* work; and, as I am preparing for publication another which will treat exclusively of impediments of speech, I shall conclude the present chapter with the following

Remarks on Stammering, from a Lecture on Elocution, delivered before the American Lyceum, May 6, 1837, by Andrew Comstock, M.D.

For the last ten years the author of these REMARKS has been engaged in an investigation of the philosophy of the human voice, with a view to the formation of a system of just Elocution, and to the discovery of the true means for removing IMPEDIMENTS OF SPEECH IN STAMMERERS. How far he has succeeded in his attempt, is not for him to say. His system is the result of his own reflection and experience; and, as it is founded in philosophy, it is the only *true* system. The following pages contain the mere outlines of the system. The work itself will be presented to the public as soon as the author's other labours will permit.

Stammering or stuttering is a hesitation or interruption of speech, and is usually attended with more or less distortion of feature. This affection presents itself under a variety of forms; but my limits will not allow me to give a particular description of them. I will notice only the most striking.

In some cases, the stammerer makes an effort to speak, and all his breath is expelled without producing vocality; in others, the lips are spasmodically closed:—these two forms often occur in the same case. Sometimes the stammerer, while speaking or reading, loses all power over the vocal organs, and remains some moments with his mouth open, before he can recover sufficient energy to proceed. In many cases, the stammerer repeats the word immediately preceding the one he is attempting to pronounce, or he repeats, in a rapid manner, the first element, or the first syllable, of the difficult word.

CAUSES.—The predisposing causes are nervous irritability and delicacy of constitution.

The most usual *exciting* causes are diffidence, embarrassment, a fear of not being successful when about to make an effort to speak, an attempt to speak faster than the vocal organs can assume the proper positions for utterance. Two or more of these causes often occur in the same case. Sometimes the habit of stammering is acquired by imitation.

The *proximate* cause of stammering is a spasmodic action of the muscles of speech.

PROGNOSIS.—The probability of a cure depends upon the following circumstances: If the stammerer has a cheerful disposition, is distinguished for energy of mind and decision of character, can appreciate the variations of pitch in speech and song, or, in other words, has an ear for music and a taste for elocution, the prognosis is favourable. But if he is of a nervous temperament, subject to melancholy, irresolute of purpose, incapable of imitation in speaking and singing, the prognosis is unfavourable.

TREATMENT.—The stammerer should be impressed with the importance, nay, necessity, of giving exclusive attention to the subject; and he should not be allowed to converse with any one till he can speak without stammering. These rules cannot be too strongly enforced. I am fully persuaded of this from my own experience. Several stammerers, who have placed themselves under my care, taking but two or three lessons a week and attending to their usual avocations, have left me disappointed; while those who have given undivided attention to the subject, have been entirely relieved. True, many are more or less benefited even by occasionally taking a lesson; but it is very difficult, by any irregular course, to effect a radical cure. The habit of stammering should be arrested at once; for, while it is continued, how is it possible that the habit of speaking correctly can be established?

Great pains should be taken to inspire the stammerer with confidence. He should be convinced that his success depends mainly upon his own exertions: that he must pursue the various exercises assigned him with indefatigable zeal, with untiring industry; that he has the same organs of speech as other people, and nothing is necessary to enable him to use them as well, but a conviction in his ability to do so. To think that one *can* do, gives almost the ability to accomplish——but to think that one *cannot* do, virtually takes away the ability to do, even where it is ample.

Stammering is often continued by the subordinate estimation which the stammerer puts upon himself. He is too apt to consider those around him giants, and himself a dwarf. As this estimation of himself serves to perpetuate his disease, it is clear that its remedy must be found in making himself equal to any: if this mental classification into giants and dwarfs must take place, let the stammerers make themselves the giants, and those around them the dwarfs.

The teacher should study the disposition of his pupil: he should persuade him to banish from his mind all melancholy thoughts—in short, he should do every thing in his power to render his pupil cheerful and happy.

Various athletic exercises should be resorted to daily, to invigorate all the muscles of voluntary motion, and diminish nervous irritability. In some cases it may be necessary to have recourse to tonics, anti-spasmodics, bathing in salt water, frictions over the whole surface of the body, &c., &c. Electricity may be used with advantage as a tonic, and also as a means of interrupting the spasm of the vocal organs.

The vocal treatment is deduced from the following circumstances:

(1) An ability to sing.

(2) An ability to speak when alone:

(3) And if the stammerer must speak before an audience, the smaller the audience and the farther he is removed from it, the better.

(4) An ability to speak amidst a noise that is sufficient to render the human voice nearly or quite inaudible.

(5) An ability to speak better in the dark than in the light.

(6) An ability to speak in a measured manner.

(7) An ability to speak in a drawling manner.

(8) An ability to speak with the mouth more or less distorted.

(9) An ability to speak in any key, either higher or lower than that in which the stammerer usually converses.

(10) An ability to speak with a halloo.

(1) An ability to speak when the attention is divided or arrested by some object or circumstance more or less irelevant to the subject.

(12) An ability to speak in concert or simultaneously. Every one who has learned to sing, knows how much easier it is to sing in concert than alone. All the exercises, therefore, for the cure of stammering, should, at first, be conducted in concert.

Stammering may be considered a fault in elocution, the result of defective education, and is confirmed by habit. If children were properly instructed in speaking and reading, this affection of the vocal organs would, probably, seldom or never occur. Hence, no mode of treatment that is not founded in just elocution or the correct exercise of the organs of speech for the purposes of vocal expression, can be relied on. This must appear obvious to every intelligent and reflecting mind. The stammerer must be taught how to give language the pitch, time, and force which the sense requires. To effect this, his muscles of speech, which have long been refractory, must be trained till they are brought under the control of volition, and like a well-marshalled troop of soldiers, made to act in harmonious concert.

Oral language may be resolved into certain sounds which are its elements. Now there are certain positions of the organs of speech more favourable than others for the production of the elements. The stammerer should be made thoroughly acquainted with these positions, and, in connexion with them, should be required to exercise his voice in the most energetic manner upon all the elements singly, till he can utter them without hesitation. He should also utter them in various combinations, not only according to the laws of syllabication, but in every irregular way. The vowels should be exploded from the throat with great force; and they should be sung, as well as pronounced with the rising and falling inflection, through every interval of pitch within the compass of the voice.

The pupil should be drilled in various exercises whose highest peculiarity is time and force. Time may be measured by means of the Metronome, by beating with the hand, and by marching.[1] Pitch, time, and force, are the elements of expression, and a proper combination of them in reading and speaking, constitutes good elocution. When, therefore, the stammerer becomes master of these elements, as well as the elements of the language, he may commence speaking and reading. In his first attempts at conversation, both teacher and pupil should speak in a deliberate manner, with a full, firm tone of voice, and in a very low pitch.

The stammerer should now commit to memory a short piece which requires to be spoken with explosive force; for example, ''Satan's speech to his legions.'' The members of the class should stand at a sufficient distance from each other to prevent their hands coming in contact when their arms are extended. They should then pronounce the speech in concert, after the teacher, and accompany it with appropriate gesticulation. It should be repeated again and again, till each pupil can give it proper expression, both as regards voice and gesture. Each pupil should then, in turn, take the place of the teacher and give out the speech to the class. To prevent the pupil's stammering, while he is performing the teacher's part, the teacher himself should play an accompaniment on the violoncello, violin, organ, drum, or some other instrument. At first the notes should be made very loud; but if the effort of the pupil, standing out of the class, is likely to be successful, they should gradually be made softer and softer, and, finally, the accompaniment omitted altogether. This piece should be pronounced alternately with one which requires to be spoken with long quantity and in a low pitch, as ''Ossian's Address to the Sun.''

When the pupil has mastered these two kinds of reading, he may take up dignified dialogue, and, lastly, conversational pieces. He should drawl out

---

[1] Also by beating with the dumb-bells.

difficult words, which are generally those having short vowels preceded by labials, dentals, and gutturals.

In very bad cases of stammering, the pupil should first sing the words, then drawl them, then pronounce them with very long quantity, and thus gradually approximate to common speaking.

As soon as the pupils can speak without stammering, they should recite singly in a very large room, or in the open air, at a distance from the audience, which, at first, should consist of the members of the class only. A few visitors should be occasionally introduced, and the number should be gradually increased. In this way the stammerer will soon acquire sufficient confidence to speak before a large assembly. In some cases it may be expedient for the stammerer to recite before an audience in a dark room; but as he acquires confidence, light should be gradually admitted.

Stammerers, instead of speaking immediately after inspiration, as they should do, often attempt to speak immediately after expiration, when, of course, they have no power to speak. The lungs, like a bellows, perform their part in the process of speaking, best, when plentifully supplied with air. This is an important fact, and should be remembered, not only by stammerers, but also by those who have occasion to read or speak in public. Loud speaking, long-continued, with the lungs but partially distended, is very injurious to these organs: it is apt to occasion a spitting of blood, which is not unfrequently a precursor of pulmonary consumption. But loud speaking, with proper management of the breath, is a healthful exercise: besides strengthening the muscles which it calls into action, it promotes the decarbonization of the blood, and, consequently, exerts a salutary influence on the system generally.

A facsimile of the original title page of this work is reproduced on p. 158.

A SYSTEM

OF

E L O C U T I O N,

WITH

SPECIAL REFERENCE

TO

G E S T U R E,

TO THE TREATMENT OF

STAMMERING,

AND

DEFECTIVE ARTICULATION,

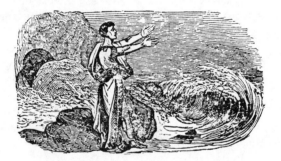

COMPRISING NUMEROUS DIAGRAMS, AND ENGRAVED
FIGURES, ILLUSTRATIVE OF THE SUBJECT.

BY ANDREW COMSTOCK, M. D.

Can Elocution be taught? This question has heretofore been asked through ignorance.
It shall hereafter be asked, only through folly. *Rush's Philosophy of the Human Voice.*

PHILADELPHIA:
PUBLISHED BY THE AUTHOR.
VOCAL GYMNASIUM, FOURTH STREET ABOVE CHESTNUT—
DWELLING HOUSE, No. 100 MULBERRY STREET.
1841.

Remarks on Stammering, from the
American Journal of Medical Science,
Vol. 21, Pages 75–99, Philadelphia, 1837

A physician who has had an opportunity of observing a chronic disease in his own person, may naturally be supposed better qualified to write upon that disease, than one whose attention has only been called to the matter he treats upon, in the common routine of practice. Lancisi, Corvisart, Bayle, Laennec, Floyer and Bree, were victims of the diseases upon which they have given us so much information. This consideration has led me to suppose I might perform a useful service in committing to paper some remarks, the result of my experience, upon the subject of Psellismus.

The obscurity which rests upon it, and the vague and conjectural manner in which most medical writers are content to treat it, is matter of much surprise. The hesitation and doubt, on the one hand, with which professional writers allude to it; and, on the other hand, the confidence with which the inventors of systems for its cure set forth their claims, are equally remarkable. It seems evident that the subject has obtained very little attention from physicians.

A desire is constantly expressed by reviewers and journalists, as well as by the profession at large, that persons who undertake to write upon impediments of speech, upon the organs of articulation, or upon the art of speaking, would throw more light upon the mechanism of the human voice. It is supposed that if this mechanism were well understood, the manner of correcting its defects would be rendered easy.

If our watch is out of order, if it will not keep time, if the hand will not move in accordance with the action of the spring, we must make ourselves acquainted with its intimate structure before we can rectify the defect.

This reasoning, but for one objection, would apply exactly to the human body—to the human voice. We must understand the machinery; we must know whether the defect is in the nerves, the arteries, the muscles, the skin, or the alimentary canal, before we can prescribe. There is only one thing wanting to make the analogy complete. This is, that however clearly we may make ourselves acquainted with the machinery, i.e., the anatomy and physiology of the human body, there is one thing we cannot understand. The spring is invisible—the manner in which it acts is unknown.

Whatever knowledge discoveries in anatomy and surgery may give us of the organs of speech, no light will be thrown upon the means of remedying the impediment. Why? Simply because the organs may be perfect, and yet the speech defective. In the majority of stammerers there is no organic defect.

As well might we expect to cure an epileptic patient by explaining to him the nature of muscular power, informing him that the muscles are stimulated to contract through the medium of certain nerves; that these nerves may be traced to the spinal cord, and this to the brain. Here we have the whole machinery well known. Skin, muscle, bone, nerves, and blood-vessels, are all known; and, as far as we can see, are perfect. In ordinary cases, we will to move our hand, and our hand moves; and it does not move but by our will. The case with our patient is simply reversed; he wills to move his hand, and it does *not* move, or its motions are beyond his control.

It is the same with the stammerer. He wills to utter an articulate sound, but the sound does not come; *vox faucibus haesit*. In cases an inarticulate sound is produced, the actions of the facial muscles and the jaw are irregular and spasmodic, producing distortion of the features, while the emission of sound not being in accordance with, and consequently not modulated by, the action of the muscles of articulation, may even become a howl.

If I am asked how it can be proved that there is no defect in the organs of speech of the stammerer, I answer, because if you place him in certain circumstances, his speech will become perfectly free. Organic defects are known by the constancy of their symptoms. It is a well known fact that most, if not all, stammerers, can sing with ease. Most of them can read poetry fluently. Some are entirely free from their impediment when by themselves. They can speak or read aloud for hours when they know no one hears them, without the slightest hesitation or catch in their voice. Perhaps they can read or speak with more fluency than those who have no impediment; for those who are led by this defect to pay great attention to the means of acquiring a free and faultless mode of speech, will, when free from it, be better speakers than those whose attention has never been called to the subject of elocution. It is a fact, though but little noticed, except by teachers of elocution and those who have been led to observe particularly the conversation of others, that perfectly easy and fluent speech is rare; at least among the male part of society. A stammerer who is perfectly cured will be a better speaker than is generally met with, for all the means for overcoming stammering are adapted to produce fluent and faultless speech.

If stammerers, then, can, under certain circumstances, speak thus fluently, does it not prove that there is no defect in the organs. Were stammering produced by a defect in the organs of articulation and voice, the subject would continue to stammer under all circumstances. The mere removal from an occupied to an unoccupied apartment would make no difference; it could not restore parts that were deficient, nor remove parts that were redundant.

That there are defects of speech produced by organic disease, I am well aware; but in general these may be ascertained by inspection of the organs. Thus, the removal of the tongue, the loss of teeth, harelip, and, above all, fissure of the palate, may produce imperfect or inarticulate utterance of the worst kind. These causes, however, do not produce stammering.

If there is, therefore, no organic defect,—if the patient can speak freely when alone, and if the mere presence of another person causes him to stammer,—does it not prove that his impediment is owing solely to mental causes; that his is a mental affection?

Stammering, however, is a complicated affection. It originates in weakness of the nervous system—in irregular action of the nerves. Afterwards, the fear of stammering causes a person to stammer; the organs of speech soon acquire a depraved habit; the nerves also are habituated to irregular action, as in chorea, and the habit may become difficult to eradicate, even if the mental cause is removed. We have, therefore, mental and physical causes united, in every degree of complication.

The mental emotion increases the effect produced by the vicious habit of the organs, and this habit increases the mental emotion. Thus, these two causes are constantly acting on each other and aggravating the disease. Some persons never allow the fear of stammering to prevent the expression of their thoughts; but others acquire habits of silence, and of thinking so much before they speak, that they lose the power of translating their thoughts readily into tangible words, if I may use the expression, and hence the want of command of language is added to their other difficulties. An habitual stammerer of this kind, if suddenly relieved from his impediment, will find almost as much difficulty from this want of command of words as he did before from his defect of utterance. There is also another difficulty, which is, that his attention being always divided between the words he has to utter, and the consideration how he is to utter them, his ideas become confused, and very probably he forgets the latter part of his sentence before he has uttered the first. If mental embarrassment of any kind, if want of a perfect coolness and knowledge of what he is to say, will make a good public speaker stammer, it may be understood in how much greater degree it will operate to increase a habit of stammering. I may allude to another thing also, which gives a singular appearance to the conversation of the stammerer, even when he appears to speak with ease. This is, that without being perfectly aware of it himself, he is constantly considering before he speaks, whether the words he means to employ are easy to articulate; and he is constantly in search of easy words. Hence, he makes use of odd and outrè expressions; and as no two words are perfectly synonymous, the words he substitutes for those which would more perfectly express his meaning, and which are chosen in haste, and for no other reason than easy utterance, often sound odd, or convey a meaning very different from what he wishes. Although he may see that this is the case, yet exhausted by the effort he has already made, he does not attempt to correct the impression he has communicated. In this way he may very readily obtain the character of an idiot or an imbecile.

I have spoken of stammering as the result of derangement of the nervous system. It is so often said to be produced by imitation, that some further remarks on this head may be necessary. I cannot pretend to bring the numerical system to my aid —I cannot exactly say how many out of a hundred stammerers are of the sanguine or the athletic temperament, but this I will affirm, that having had ample opportunity of observing numbers of persons thus affected, I believe an athletic, sanguine, or a phlegmatic stammerer to be very rare. The affection occurs in persons of extreme susceptibility, whose constitutions would readily make them the subjects of hysteria or chorea. This nervous susceptibility may be caused by sickness in childhood. This is the remote cause.

One exciting cause may be this, that persons who are thus susceptible may be so readily carried away by strong feelings, that in the hurry and earnestness to express their ideas, they crowd their words so rapidly upon each other as to produce stammering. They are constantly the subjects of those ardent emotions, that are occasional causes of stammering in good speakers. *This is not a place for me* to discuss the connexion between thought and words, otherwise I might prove that the time required for the articulation of a single word, is sufficient for a long train of thought to pass through the mind. *Now, the earnest endeavour to express thoughts as rapidly as they are conceived, will produce stammering. This is what we often witness in persons who are not stammerers.*

Fear is often an exciting cause of stammering. A child of the constitutional susceptibility spoken of above, may be made a stammerer by bad treatment. If he is in constant awe of a brutal parent or master, this is a sufficient cause. In regard to imitation as a cause, I believe it to be comparatively rare. From the known tendency of chorea and hysteria to be extended by imitation, we might imagine this to be a more frequent cause than it actually is.

It is not my present purpose to write a detailed or a systematic treatise upon impediments of speech; I design, merely, to offer a few hints upon a subject which appears to have been little investigated by medical men, and which is certainly very little understood.

An extract from a letter of Richard Cull, quoted in the Medico-Chirurgical Review, for October, 1836, may serve to give an idea of the present state of medical knowledge on this subject.

It would be tedious to enumerate the various methods that ignorance, empiricism and imposture have, at various times, proposed for the cure of impediments of speech. From the farmer in Joe Miller, who made his son sing 'Daddy your house is on fire,' down to Mrs. Leigh, the lady in New York, who forces her disciples to keep the tongue against the teeth uninterruptedly for three days, the plans have been innumerable, the proposers confident, and the success, of course, immense. Yet, singular as it would seem, although each is perfectly successful, the one that follows is advanced expressly because no such thing as success can be obtained. How this paradoxical state of things may be explained we leave to others to determine.

Of Mrs. Leigh's system, and the above amusing misrepresentation of it, I will speak hereafter.

There are two different species of stammering, which I shall describe. The first is that in which the organs of articulation, the lips and tongue are concerned. In the second, the organs are not in fault, but the voice is wanting. The effort to speak is made, the lips and tongue move, but the voice will not come. A person who witnesses this attempt, will believe that the individual has spoken, and ask him to repeat what he has said. The two kinds are frequently united. Indeed, when the voice is not at the command of the patient, the violent efforts he makes to speak will produce convulsive motions of the features and distortion of the countenance. A habit will be formed by the nerves and muscles, and these irregular motions will afterward take place, even when the voice is under command. A paroxysm of stammering is truly formidable to witness. The countenance of the patient is horribly distorted, inarticulate and dissonant sounds issue from his mouth; he will tear his hair, stamp as if with rage, and practise all the gestures of a madman. Even in less violent cases, the whole nervous system is in intense agitation, every nerve in his body, to the ends of his fingers and his toes, seems to him to vibrate, like the strings of a harp, producing a sensation like that caused by the filing of a saw, and he feels a sense of suffocation at his chest. I may mention, incidently, that stammerers are said, in general, to have narrow chests, and that their lungs have not free play. My experience as far as it goes, confirms this. A narrow chest also, is said to be one of the characteristics of the nervous temperament. I have seen some athletic stammerers, at least one or two, but the most I have seen belong to the nervous class.

The first species is what is properly called stammering, and consists in the simple repetition of the same sound over and over, attended with convulsive motions of the lips, tongue, and muscles of the face. This is infinitely more disagreeable, and apparently worse than the other. It is, however, much more readily cured. The second species is more purely dependent upon an affection of the mind than the first. I think it in general, if not always, is the result of the first species. The fear of stammering produces that embarrassment which causes the voice to fail, either by closing the glottis, or by causing the patient to inhale when he ought to exhale.

It is well known that singers, when embarrassed, are incapable of uttering a single note; their voice is gone. In the same manner, a speaker before a public assembly sometimes loses his voice; and the more anxious he is to speak—the greater exertion he makes—the more totally unable is he to bring forth a sound. The more powerful passions, also, such as grief, fear, anger, and even excessive joy, completely take away the power of utterance. They not only, in many cases, deprive the subject, of the power of distinct articulation, but even of the ability to produce a sound: the vocal passage is spasmodically closed. Thus a person is said to be choked with rage. The same passions, in a less degree, will produce the first species of stammering in persons whose ordinary utterance is fluent.

I may be asked, if singers are thus subject to loss of voice, why does not the same thing oftener occur in regard to speech? I answer, because singing is merely an accomplishment; it is acquired by study and effort; whereas speech is in general so early learnt, that it may be almost considered spontaneous. Men talk without previously considering in what manner they are to move their lips, where the voice is to come from, how the sound is to be produced, or what organs are to be set in motion. A man wills to move his arms, his arm moves; he wills to speak, and the words are uttered: one is as little the object of thought as the other. I may here remark, too, a curious fact; that it is impossible for a stammerer to stammer by design. Desire him to stammer; let him make the attempt, and he will speak as freely as any one. Of course I do not refer to those stammerers of the first species, the vicious habit of whose organs is so confirmed that they can never articulate without stammering. This, however, is a rare case.

But let us alter the natural order of things. Suppose we could make speech as much a matter of education as singing. Let us take a young person of considerable susceptibility; impress upon his mind the idea that speech is a subject that requires great thought; that it is of vast importance for him to educate his voice and his organs of articulation; and very probably when you introduce him into company, his voice will utterly fail. I have already said that I believe an impediment of the second kind to be the sequel of the first. A child is afflicted with stammering, and the constant and unsuccessful efforts made to overcome the defect, produce so powerful an effect on his mind, that whenever he attempts to speak, the fear of stammering, the constant thought as to how he is to speak, the constant dread of failure, deprives him of voice. Parents may learn from this the extreme necessity which exists for caution in subjecting a child who stammers to a variety of methods for its relief. No trial should be made at home. An experienced person should be selected to make the trial. I mean the person, if any such can be found, who has had the greatest experience in the treatment of defects of speech: and if none such can be found, or if, after a reasonable length of time, the trial fails, none other should ever be made. And this caution should be kept in mind: that in subjecting the child to a course of treatment for the removal of the defect, you fix the matter so much in his mind, that if not relieved, it will be aggravated and confirmed.

But to return to the analogy of singing—we have then only to make speech as much a matter of education, as much an accomplishment as singing, and the performers will be as liable to loss of voice, when embarrassed, as singers. Of course there would be the same difference between the bold and confident and the diffident and reserved, in the one case as in the other. Many persons may find it difficult to conceive that they could, under any circumstances, be thus deprived of the power of speech. But these same bold speakers, if possessed of musical powers, would be equally bold singers.

It is well known that a single idea, constantly dwelt upon, produces madness: in like manner, the idea of the importance of correcting a bad habit of speech may be carried so far as to become *a monomania.* Thelwall, who has given, I think, a very accurate description of the varieties of impediments of speech, says that there are some forms which bear a close relation to mental derangement. This remark may be still further strengthened by the instances of those defects of articulation produced by blows on the head.

I have made a reference to Mr. Thelwall's letter, and also a quotation from Mr. Cull's. The latter alludes to the numerous methods of cure which have been represented by their authors as completely successful, and all of which seem to have failed. From the knowledge of the subject that Mr. Thelwall exhibits, I have no doubt of his ability in the cure of impediments of speech. I believe that there are now many persons who have devoted themselves to the observation and treatment of this defect, who are capable of curing it. One principal reason that many of the cures are not permanent is, that the teachers require too little time. A habit that has been confirmed by years cannot be eradicated in a few weeks. The best musical teachers now inform their pupils that the art of singing requires years of practice and instruction. In the same manner does it require years of practice under the direction of a competent instructor, for a stammerer to acquire the free use of speech. The same thing that occurs in other chronic diseases takes place in this. A patient applies to us for the cure of distorted spine. He is told that he cannot be cured under a year. After pursuing the proper course for three months, he finds himself very much benefitted. Having now acquired the habit of using the various machines with facility, and convinced that the means prescribed will complete his cure, he requests our permission to return into the country. The country air will be beneficial to him; he can carry his weights, his pulleys, his triangle, and all his other apparatus with him. He arrives at home, and amid the excitement of meeting his friends, and the exhilaration produced by their congratulations on his amendment, his exercises are neglected. A few days or a few weeks can make no difference; time passes, and the longer he neglects it the greater is his reluctance to resume the wearisome course he formerly pursued. By and by, he finds the disease once more making progress, and now very probably he loses confidence in his surgeon, and in the course he formerly thought so successful. It is the same in other chronic diseases. What physician is there who does not feel that the moment his inspection is removed, the rules he has laid down will probably be pursued with less energy than before? But ought this to bring discredit upon the physician, or upon the means employed? Certainly not.

The cure of impediments of speech is now much better understood, by those who have devoted themselves to their treatment, than it was twenty years ago, at least in this country. Mr. Thelwall's letter, and his *Results of Experience,* were published in London in 1810 and 1814, and although there can be no doubt that he performed the cures he describes, yet his book throws no light on the subject. Having much experience of the methods formerly resorted to, and which were in fact merely experimental, I can affirm that many of them were more calculated to confirm than to eradicate the defect.

Despite of all the ridicule that has been cast upon Mrs. Leigh's system, by those who knew nothing about it, I believe the inventor of this system deserves the credit of the improvement. As it was at first taught empirically, the pupils being obliged to take an oath not to reveal the secret, many amusing misconceptions arose in regard to it; the pupils often purposely misleading those who subjected them to troublesome inquiries. Hence arose the brilliant discovery that was published in our daily papers at the time when it was taught in Boston by Mr. Wilson. I mean the discovery that the system consisted in obliging the pupils to keep their tongue in contact with their teeth three days in succession.

Mrs. Leigh's system exceeded all others in the marvellous rapidity with which the cures were wrought, and it was this very incredible rapidity that brought ridicule upon the system. Anything that gives a system the appearance of the marvellous, is sufficient, in our day, to cause its rejection. Yet the phenomena of the human mind are no better understood than they were formerly. There is a practical disbelief with regard to the existence of mind, but still its action upon the body cannot be at all understood. We are every now and then meeting with instances of this action of the mind or the imagination upon the system which are, to all appearance, miraculous. But, to put the power of the imagination out of the question for the present, the apparent miraculousness of these cures disappears when the system is understood.

A deaf person may be made to hear instantaneously by giving him an ear trumpet; in like manner a person may be made to talk freely by telling him how to talk. I am well acquainted with a gentleman who formerly stammered as much as an individual could do, and in the way most disagreeable to witness. He was cured in half an hour. He required, it is true, superintendence for some time afterwards, but he was always a rapid speaker; and though he formerly stammered most furiously with lip and tongue, his defect never made him refrain from speaking. The consequence was, that the moment he was put in possession of a mode of speaking freely, his words flowed forth with the utmost volubility. Though it is now some years since his cure, his impediment has never returned; and neither in private or in company can any difficulty be observed in his utterance. Other patients were cured as rapidly, and in some cases the cure was permanent. In many cases, however, the patient on his return home gradually relapsed into his former condition.

References

The [1] inventor of Mrs. Leigh's system, (for Mrs. Leigh was not the inventor) a medical gentleman of high talents and very strong natural powers, had a daughter afflicted with stammering. After attentive observation and long study of her case, he succeeded in hitting upon a method which effected a cure. This method was imparted to the young lady's instructress, Mrs. Leigh, an Englishwoman, in order that it might be pursued during school hours.

---

[1]Dr. Christopher C. Yates, of New York.

The inventor soon determined to extend its benefits to others. Finding Mrs. Leigh enter into the scheme with zeal and ability, he placed her at the head of the institution; and fearful of the reproach of empiricism, he chose it should pass under her name. Pupils soon flocked to them, they acquired experience and brought their system to perfection. The marvellous rapidity of the cures brought them immense numbers. It would not have seemed possible that what appears to be a rare defect should have proved to be shared by so many. They soon found it expedient to qualify other teachers, who established themselves in all parts of the union. Mr. Wilson, a very intelligent young man of unwearied industry, taught the system some time in Boston. The results here, as in New York, appeared wonderful; and if they were not permanent, the fault was in the short time allowed for the cure. The time Mr. Wilson fixed was six weeks, but many of the pupils believing themselves cured, remained not half that time.

Two great mistakes were undoubtedly committed. The first was, in attempting to make permanent cures in so short a time. The second was, in attempting to qualify so many teachers. Most of them, probably, believed that the possession of the secret was all that was requisite. They were not aware that years of observation and experience, a knowledge of elocution, a knowledge of the human mind and of human nature, were requisite to make them successful teachers. It is the same with this as with other diseases. If we had certain remedies for certain diseases—if for instance a certain dose of calomel would cure every case of fever, the science of medicine would be perfectly simple, and might be practised by a child. But the skilful physician adapts his remedies to the particular constitution of his patient, and to the greater or less development of particular symptoms. It is symptoms he is called to combat, and the symptoms in no two cases are the same. Now the power to do this is only to be acquired by attentive observation and experience. This remark applies with still greater force to impediments of speech. In the treatment of no other complaint is experience more essential than in this. I need not mention also, that unwearied industry and patience are requisite on the part of the teacher as well as on that of the pupil. This fact may afford some light as to the reason why a method successful in the hands of the inventor generally fails in the hands of others. No methods invented for the cure of stammering, have met with general success, because such methods are incommunicable, at least by writing. A successful teacher may be able to communicate his art to another of sufficient intelligence and industry, but it cannot be done at once, any more than a man ignorant of music can become qualified by a single lesson to teach music.

The gentleman who invented Mrs. Leigh's system was qualified for the purpose as few men can be. Not destitute of sufficient learning, he has yet little reliance on books, and depends upon observation, principally, for his sources of knowledge. Possessed of a tall and commanding figure, with an air of confidence and decision, he inspires his pupil at once with perfect confidence. He tells his patient *how* to speak; he tells him he *can* speak; and he *does* speak.

The effect of imparting their method to so many teachers, was soon apparent.

The cures obtained were so numerous and wonderful, and attended with so much profit to the teachers, that multitudes of other persons soon set up to cure impediments of speech. It is not surprising, therefore, that the system soon fell into disrepute.

The inventor, at first, gave directions merely for the position of the tongue, but afterwards he made great improvement in his treatment. The suppression of the voice he believed to be caused by a spasmodic closure of the glottis, the same cause to which Dr. Arnott ascribes stammering.[2] The patient, in his violent and ill directed efforts to speak, closes the glottis, and hence the sound cannot escape. He makes motions with his lips and tongue, but the more violent his efforts, the more firmly is the glottis closed. The object of first importance, therefore, is to get the glottis open, the next is to keep it so.

The foundation of all rational systems taught for the relief of stammering, are based upon two well known facts. The first is, that slowness and deliberation are requisite for perfect speech. The second fact is, that stammerers can sing with great facility. In singing the sound is continued from syllable to syllable, and word to word, more than in common speech; there is less emphasis, less interruption of sound. Hints have been taken from this fact, and various methods invented to prolong the sound in this manner, and prevent its interruption until the speaker arrives at the end of his sentence. So long as the stammerer can prolong the sound in this way, he can speak with ease; his great difficulty is in the commencement of a sentence and in avoiding interruption in breaking the sound into syllables.

An attention to the patient's manner of inspiration is, therefore, of importance. Instructions are given for inhaling with deliberation, and for husbanding the breath, so as to let it out no faster than is requisite for the formation of sound, and without panting or any sudden or spasmodic effort. Directions must also be given as to the particular manner in which each consonant is pronounced, and for the articulation of any particular words or sounds which are difficult to the pupil. These must be taught, and any vicious pronunciation corrected by precept and example. For this purpose, an acquaintance with the principles of elocution, and with elementary sounds, is requisite. It is by imitation only that the proper manner of uttering them is to be acquired, and the organs habituated to it.

Mr. King, the teacher of elocution, who gave lessons in Boston in 1835, for the cure of stammering, was well qualified in this respect from his knowledge of elocution, in which he was an able instructer. This, and his experience in the treatment of impediments of speech, rendered him a very competent teacher. I believe his method to be adequate to the cure, if pursued with sufficient attention and perseverance, and for sufficient time. Mr. King's system requires more labour

---

[2]Dr. Arnott, in his work on physics, considers stammering in every case produced by spasmodic closure of the glottis. Dr. Yates holds the same opinion; and it is remarkable if, as I believe to be the case, the opinion of each was formed from his own observation and was original with both.

on the part both of teacher and pupil than Mrs. Leigh's. He aims less at producing rapid and striking results. But he puts into the hands of his pupils certain rules, which, when they have attained proficiency in them by imitation and practice, will enable them to cure themselves with perfect certainty, if they are not wanting in perseverance. In this respect, the system is more tangible than Mrs. Leigh's. It is more capable of being continued after the pupil is deprived of the aid and superintendence of the teacher. Mr. King assigned one year as the shortest time in which the defect can be eradicated. He did not, however, require that the pupil should remain all this time under his inspection.

According to Mrs. Leigh's system, the pupil was kept in the house of the instructer, so as to be under his eye during nearly the whole time; so that he was made conversant with the method in less time than by Mr. King's course, who gave lessons of one hour a day. Now it will be much better for the pupil, especially if an adult, to receive instruction for an hour a day for a year, than to be with the instructer the whole time for a fortnight. For children, the best plan would be for them to be with the instructer all the time during two, four, or six weeks, according to circumstances, and afterwards receive an hour's instruction daily for a year. Of course it is not to be expected that this hour daily will be sufficient; the pupil must practise by himself several hours, and he will do this more regularly while he continues to take lessons, and will also avoid errors in his practise which an individual, whether child or adult, will insensibly fall into, if left entirely to himself.

Dr. M'Cormac of Edinburgh, published a treatise on the cure of stammering in 1828. The following quotation, from his preface, appears on his title page.

> I can assure all, that by the most ordinary attention to the following pages, they may of themselves remove, with the utmost ease and facility, and in a very short space of time, the most inveterate and confirmed habits of stuttering, no matter of how many years duration or when contracted.

This is being pretty confident. Dr. M'Cormac's observations, however, do not appear to be the results of experience; his treatise has never obtained much attention, and I do not know that since he published it, he has ever added or improved what was then mere theory. If he had tested it, by devoting himself to the cure of stammering, it is highly probable he would have become very successful. Experience would have led him to modify his theory very essentially. As it is, his treatise fails in the object aimed at, because defects of speech cannot be cured by a book. We cannot learn to sing from a book, neither can we learn to speak. A stammerer learning to speak is exactly in the position of a person learning to sing. A singing master can teach a pupil of sufficient industry to sing, and a person experienced in the treatment of impediments of speech can teach his pupil to speak freely and well, provided sufficient time and pains be taken.

It seems that, while travelling in America some years since, Dr. M'Cormac's attention was attracted by the well confirmed success of Mrs. Leigh's system, which was then taught under oath of secrecy at New York.

The desire that results so beneficial should be placed within the reach of every one, led him to reflect much upon the causes of stammering, and he finally came to the conclusion that the "proximate cause in most cases *arises from the patient endeavoring to utter words, or any other manifestation of voice, when the air in the lungs is exhausted, and they are in a state of collapse, or nearly so.*" This is the discovery upon which he rests his claim, and this is the foundation of his system. But, if what I have said above be true, it will be seen that this is only one form of stammering. The vicious habit of the articulating organs may exist independently of any deficiency of voice. Dr. M'Cormac's directions for inhaling, if practised upon, are more likely to lead the patient astray and to confirm a bad habit of inhalation, or produce one equally bad, than to remedy the difficulty. Without doubt an attention to the manner of inhalation, where the voice is in fault, is of the first importance; means must be taken to keep the air passages open, and to prevent any attempt at speech with the lungs in a state of collapse. If the person attempts utterance by inspiration instead of expiration, he will succeed only in producing with great difficulty a monosyllable, and the effort will be attended with great exhaustion. I do not see that it makes much difference whether we describe this as an attempt to speak with the lungs collapsed, or with the glottis spasmodically closed. The simple fact is, that the breath is not expired at the proper moment to produce articulate sound, and it is emitted in irregular jets. The patient must therefore be taught to respire slowly, regularly, and without effort. Dr. M'Cormac says also, and truly, that the patient having acquired a vicious habit of utterance, he must be carried back to the beginning, and taught to speak entirely over again. Unfortunately, he has not only to learn to speak anew, but he has to unlearn a bad habit of speaking. Herein is the almost absolute necessity of a teacher, or at least an assistant. The vowel sounds are generally uttered without difficulty by the stammerer; they come from the throat without any action of the muscles of articulation, and hence they come out with ease. The difficulty is with the consonants. It is therefore necessary for the stammerer to have some one with him to remind him of every vicious attempt at speech, and to show him by example how the sounds are articulated, the position of the organs, etc. This is to be learnt only by imitation. Now this practice is to be continued until the bad habit is corrected and the new one formed. Nor is the patient safe then. Until the new habit of utterance is confirmed by time, the patient is constantly in danger of a relapse. A study of the proper manner of pronouncing the elementary sounds, and an attentive observation of the defects of speech, are absolutely necessary for the teacher.

It is not my intention, however, to give a detailed account of the different methods proposed for the treatment of impediments of speech. From what I have already said, it will be seen, that *I consider it in a great measure a mental disease; perhaps I might call it a monomania.* Whatever may be the case in children, I believe it seldom continues in adults, unless kept up by mental causes. Moral remedies, therefore, are of the first importance.

It may not, however, be uninteresting to glance briefly at some of the methods formerly employed.

The best known and the most ancient of these is the Demosthenic. We are told that Demosthenes, among other means for the removal of his defective utterance, adopted the plan of speaking with pebbles in his mouth. The sanction of a great name, the well known celebrity that Demosthenes acquired as an orator, rendered this method popular. It has, therefore, been much resorted to for the cure of stammering, and various modifications have been invented. The use of pebbles, or a small piece of money held over or under the tongue, or a pea held in the mouth,—have been devised, and stammerers subjected to these processes in the course of the various experiments made upon them. M. Itard invented a platina or gold plate for this purpose, which being forked and adapted to retain its position under the tongue, could be held more conveniently than the pebbles. Now we have no account of the particular species of impediment with which the Grecian orator was affected. There is no doubt, however, that either he or his preceptor in elocution adopted the use of pebbles for the correction of some particular vice of utterance, probably in the motions of the tongue. Now it is to be recollected, as I have already stated, that the want of command over the voice, or over the organs of articulation, occasions violent and convulsive motions of all or particular organs in different persons, so that the most opposite effects are produced. Thus, some attempt to speak with their mouths stretched convulsively open, other with them spasmodically closed; some have improper habits of moving the lips; others of moving the tongue. Now, to attempt to cure a defect which does not exist, will produce the opposite defect, and even a plan wisely devised to remedy one vice, if it be persevered in after it is removed, will produce the opposite. For instance, if a stammerer who attempts to speak has his attention directed to keeping his mouth open, he will be likely, if not watched, to acquire the habit of attempting to speak with the mouth spasmodically open.

One method which I have known employed for the cure of stammering, was that of directing the pupil to press his lips firmly together, and dwell for some time upon the consonants, which he was directed to pronounce with force. This was undoubtedly devised with the idea of giving strength to weak parts: but there could not be a better plan to produce stammering, or to confirm it if it already existed.

Some stammerers are said to have been cured by learning to speak a foreign language. As the pupil in this case is required to take lessons in pronunciation, and to speak the words after his instructer, until he obtains the right sound and accent, we can easily understand how the effect is produced. If the pupil is so far interested and engaged in the acquisition of a new tongue, as to forget his impediment, he may be cured in this way; but if sensitiveness predominate, the embarrassment of endeavouring to express himself intelligibly and grammatically in a strange tongue, is added to his habitual embarrassment, and increases the difficulty in a tenfold degree.

Some instructers of schools have cured stammerers placed under their care, by calling to them the moment they begin to stammer, and obliging them to stop and commence their sentence anew. Here the same remark applies as before. The sensitive stammerer becomes confused at being thus spoken to; he forgets what he has to say, and is besides in a constant tremor for fear he shall be thus interrupted; and hence his liability to hesitate is increased.

The practice of slow and loud reading, has been generally recommended. Of the utility of this, there can be no doubt; but the attention should be directed as little as possible to the impediment.

Dr. John Bostock published in the 16th volume of the Medico-Chirurgical Transactions, an account of stammering in a plethoric subject; cured by the use of cathartics continued for eight years. The patient was a child of two or three years old when this defect of speech suddenly commenced. The effect of a cathartic was almost immediately perceptible. From the account of the case, however, it is evident, that it was more purely a disease of the nervous system, and more closely allied to chorea, than stammering usually is, and the strict diet enforced, was of more importance than the cathartics.

Learning to sing, has also been generally recommended. This must be highly beneficial, provided the sensitiveness of the pupil do not interfere here again. He must be taught to sing as an amusement merely. If he learns it as an accomplishment or as a means of cure, his voice will be liable to fail him.

Most of the methods which individuals have devised for their own cure, apply to the correction of particular defects, and should no more be used indiscriminately than calomel or venesection in every case of fever. One observation may, however, be made here, which is, that where there is not a great degree of sensitiveness, and where the patient has not already been subjected to previous experiments for his relief, any one of them may succeed merely through its influence on the imagination; or from drawing the patient's attention to the practice of the method, and diverting it from his impediment. Experiments, however, should never be made: if they do not remove, they will confirm the defect.

Having thus glanced at several of the methods of treatment proposed, I come now to the consideration of the course I judge most beneficial.

I may be asked, if I maintain the importance of an experienced teacher: can parents who have children thus afflicted, do nothing themselves? I answer that they may do almost every thing. With children, almost every thing can be done by moral treatment; and according to the moral management they meet with, will the disease be confirmed or eradicated. The subjects are generally children of extreme nervous susceptibility and of feeble constitutions. The ordinary means for producing vigour and robustness, and for strengthening the nervous system must be resorted to. The muscular system must be developed as far as possible. If the chest is narrow and contracted, every means must be employed of bringing into action the muscles of the arms and chest. For this purpose gymnastic exercises, the use of dumb bells, and various sports may be recommended. In this way, a great deal may be done to produce fulness of the chest. The child may be encouraged in the practice of these exercises as a means of acquiring physical strength, without his attention being called to his defect of speech.

As soon as he is capable of reasoning, let him be driven as much as possible into the society of other children. If his defect is laughed at, let him be habituated to bear ridicule without flinching; let him be taught that those whose feelings allow them to ridicule defects or deformities, are much more worthy of pity than the subjects of those deformities. Let him be carried to the abodes of the deaf and dumb; teach him how much happier he is than they, how great a blessing he enjoys in the use of speech, even if his speech is imperfect. Carry him also into the presence of the blind, the lame, and the deformed. Let him be familiar with the sight of those who are greater sufferers than he.

If you pursue an opposite course—if, because he is sensitive to the ridicule of other children, you let him remain at home, if you impress upon his mind the idea that he has a defect which *must* be removed, and which will be an insuperable bar to his progress in life, unless it is removed; if you allow him to perceive your constant anxiety for his cure, he will get the idea that there is something peculiar in his case—that he is marked out from mankind, as if the seal of Cain were set upon his brow; and that until he is freed from his curse, he can never associate with his fellows without shame.

On the contrary, you should direct your principal attention to convince him that his fate is not an uncommon one; that defects and diseases are the common lot, and assigned for wise purposes. In as far as you direct his attention to his defect at all, let it be with this object—to convince him that it is not an evil. Teach him resignation to the will of God. Impress upon his mind above all things, that he is under the constant protection of a being who knew what was best for him, and who has placed him in the condition and under the circumstances best adapted for his welfare. Priestly atributes the greatest blessings he enjoyed to his impediment of speech; and others may in like manner trace to the same cause, their preservation from much evil, and their possession of much happiness. Our greatest felicity is often produced by what we regard at the time as our greatest misfortunes.

When he begins to feel the importance of a free use of speech (and he may feel the importance of it without being morbidly sensitive on the subject,) and disposed to enter upon a laborious course of discipline, seek out a person who has experience in the treatment of impediments of speech. Place him under his care, and if he is benefitted, do not remove him and think to perfect the cure yourself. Recollect if one of your other children is learning to sing, you would not think of taking the task of instructer upon yourself, as soon as he had made progress. Three months is a very short time for him to remain under the superintendence of an instructer; six months is better, and where it is practicable he should remain a year. If this interferes with his other studies, it is of no consequence. He will derive benefit enough to compensate for the loss. The age I would fix upon for this trial, should be from eight to twelve. Some children, however, are as mature at the former age as others at the latter. At this period, the loss of a year's study may perchance be a gain. To a child of nervous habits, the time allowed from his instruction in speaking, may be much better employed in acquiring health and vigour, by play and exercise, than in study. But if the child is not disposed to enter into this course, if he is irritable and indocile, and regards it merely as an irksome task, it will be better to wait till a more advanced age shall convince him of its importance. Otherwise we run the risk of increasing his irritability and sensitiveness.

Should this attempt fail, none other ever ought to be made. The child should be engaged in active pursuits, and induced to be in society as much as possible. If his excessive mental susceptibility leads you into the belief that he has superior powers of mind, do not fall into the mistake of thinking that these mental powers must be cultivated. For in so doing, you are increasing his susceptibility, and rendering him miserable. The more ambitious he becomes of mental distinction, the more keen will be his sense of the defect that renders him incapable of displaying his talents and acquirements to advantage. He should be led to look forward to an active—not a literary life. He will be happier as a carpenter than as a professional man. But without resorting to a trade, there are employments enough in which he may gain wealth, and honour, (in our days we place wealth first,) and in which his impediments will be no obstacle to his success.

In very few cases, however, if the course of moral treatment I have recommended were pursued, would the complaint continue. In most cases, the moment you reconciled the mind of the patient to his defect, the moment you relieved him from the fear of stammering, he would speak freely. This is confirmed by the cases above mentioned of rapid cures produced by Mrs. Leigh's system. The patients came to the instructer fully impressed with the wonderful cures they had heard of. The appearance of the latter, his manner and voice confirmed the impression, and when he told them they could speak, they believed him, and spoke without fear, and therefore without impediment. *The mere lip and tongue stammering of children is readily cured, if the mind do not share in the disease. As they grow older they are generally capable of curing themselves.* We often meet with adults who were stammerers when children, but who cured themselves, or outgrew the disease as they acquired strength. On the other hand, adult stammerers are comparatively rare. Still more readily can the defect be removed in such cases by experienced instructers.

Moral management is, therefore, all important. In most cases it will alone be sufficient to effect a cure; and in cases where it does not, it will render the cure easy to a competent instructer. I would again urge the impropriety of subjecting the patient to a new trial if the first fails. I would urge most strenuously the necessity of leading him to the choice of that pursuit in which his defect shall afford the smallest obstacle to his progress. He is to be taught to look upon it as a necessary evil, and to shape his course accordingly. He is not to be led to bear it in his mind as the prime obstacle to his success, which must be removed before he can be happy. The molehill is thus magnified into a mountain. Whatever side he looks upon, his impediment rises up before him, shutting him out from the road to distinction. It comes to occupy so large a share of his attention that he becomes a monomaniac: on this subject, he is actually insane: there is this little diseased spot in his mind: fortunate will it be for him if it does not affect the whole; if the gangrene do not extend over all his feelings.

The characters of Lord Byron and Sir Walter Scott afford a striking illustration of the power of education to modify the effect of natural or early acquired defects, or deformities, upon the disposition. Both were the subjects of physical defects. Byron, the victim of a bad education, had been the object of various attempts to relieve this defect. This and his exposure to taunts upon the subject, fixed it in his mind, and produced a sensitiveness akin to madness. Throughout his whole life he evinces strong marks of natural benevolence and philanthropy, but he believed himself marked out from mankind, and his very best feelings turned to bitterness and misanthropy. Scott, on the contrary, whose education was very different, was rendered by his defect a more social being; more ready to enter into the feelings of those around him. It called forth his sympathy for the troubles of others. Scott was taught to bear his defect with resignation, as a necessary evil: Byron to look upon his as a disgrace which must be removed. Had Byron's feelings been soothed instead of being irritated; had he been made to witness the diseases and deformities of others, and taught how many of the same rank in life were greater sufferers than he, we might have witnessed in him all the ardour of a philanthropist. Few persons, I believe, understand how nearly philanthropy and misanthropy border on each other. The same keen sensibility, rightly directed, gives birth to the one, and wrongly directed, to the other.

> "The keenest pangs the guilty find
> Are triumph to that dreary void,
> That leafless desert of the mind,
> The waste of feelings unemployed."

It is said that Howard, if he could not have given vent to his feelings in action, would have been a madman. I will add he would at least have been a misanthrope. *Strong feelings unemployed* will turn to bitterness.

To the person whose age renders him the director of his own course, I would give the same directions. The same rules that must guide parents in the management of children, should guide him in the work of self education. *The first work the stammerer has to accomplish is the regulation of his mind;* the acquisition of perfect self command and of mental calmness. When this is done, the rest is easy. Until it is done, it is in vain for him to attempt by physical means to overcome his defect of utterance. The first embarrassment he meets with may cause its return. When he has brought himself to feel his impediment less keenly; to be less morbidly susceptible on the subject; then, if he is not already cured, let him apply to a person experienced in the treatment of stammering. If he meets, there, others who are afflicted as he is, it is all the better; he will no longer look upon his case as a peculiar one; and if he sees others whose impediments are worse than his, it will give him additional courage.

But great labour and perseverance are necessary in the employment of the physical means, in overcoming the perverse habits of the organs, and training them to articulate correctly. I would advise him, if it be possible, to pursue the method in the place of his usual residence, and while he continues his ordinary employments. An individual may leave his customary abode and pursuits, and go to a neighboring town or city for his cure. His ordinary trains of association will be broken off, and the new mode of speech will be more readily adopted while he remains absent. But the moment he returns; the moment he resumes his former avocations, and is subjected to his customary objects of anxiety, his former mode of speech returns. This difficulty, indeed, is less in proportion to the length of time allowed for the cure to become confirmed; but were this even a year, still the cure will be less permanent than if made under the circumstances by which he must be ordinarily influenced. The remarks I have made as to the length of time required for the cure of children, apply still more forcibly to the case of adults. The more confirmed the habit, the longer the time requisite for its eradication.

Dietetic and medical means may sometimes be employed by the adult with advantage. If, as is most probably the case, the patient is of a nervous temperament, means must be adopted to strengthen the nervous system, and impart vigour to the frame. No one can doubt, that in stammering, the nervous system is always more or less in fault. Now, the disorderly action of the nerves is said to be the result either of entony or atony; of too much strength or of too much weakness. In the former case, spare diet and antiphlogistic measures are necessary: in the latter, a tonic regimen.

An attention to diet is extremely important. The patient has need of all his powers of mind in their greatest vigour and clearness. He must, therefore, cautiously avoid all stimulants, even meat, unless his health requires it. The excitement produced in the system by stimulants, disposes to mental lassitude, and unfits the subject for vigorous efforts of self-discipline. Animal food in like manner, has the same effect, though in a less degree. I would not, however, recommend entire abstinence in all cases, from animal food, but only extreme moderation in diet in general, and particularly in regard to meat. This I recommend as calculated to qualify an individual for vigorous mental exertion and the possession of self command. The body must be mortified to bring it under subjection to the mind. Stimulants, moreover, excite the nervous system to irregular action. This is peculiarly the case with tobacco, and hence its use is improper. All excitement of mind or irritation of body must, in as far as is possible, be avoided or controlled. If a good speaker will stammer when under the influence of excitement, still more will an habitual stammerer.

There may be some cases in which the moderate and regular use of wine will be found beneficial; but these cases are rare, and in them the wine will be found to act as a sedative, not as a stimulant; not to produce excitement, but to check it by giving tone to the nervous system. Some persons, also, of nervous habit, may be rendered more excitable by abstinence; and their nervous system will be kept in best order by a simple but somewhat generous diet. In fine, the whole system must be kept cool by moderation, the bowels free, and every thing that excites the nervous system should be carefully avoided.

In regard to the discipline of the organs of speech, an experienced instructer, as I have repeatedly said, is of the utmost importance. *Mrs. Leigh's system is* still taught *by its inventor* in New York. That system will do all that physical instruction can do. *Mr. King's system also,* to which I have before referred, I also believe effectual. Mr. King I think now resides in *Baltimore.*

But if the patient cannot obtain such aid, what course is he to pursue? I am not sure, but what it would be best for him, to endeavour to banish the subject altogether from his mind. In regard to children, I have before alluded to the danger of subjecting them to experiments. With them it is far better, if a good teacher cannot be obtained, to attend only to the moral and physical discipline I have recommended, than to fix the idea of their defects on their minds, by trials, the results of which are altogether uncertain. A much fairer chance of relief is thus afforded them. There is one thing I might mention, which would be beneficial. Teachers of schools are apt to excuse pupils who stammer from exercises of reading and declamation; both from compassion to the unwillingness of the pupil to perform, and from the disagreeable effect on the hearers. But unless the impediment is of the worst description, it would be infinitely better for the pupil if he were induced to read and declaim with the others. It would be a useful exercise for him; it would strengthen his voice and overcome his fear of speaking before others. Besides, most stammerers can read and declaim better than they can converse. *There ought to be no distinction* of any kind made between the stammerer and other pupils.

For adults, the practice of reading aloud when alone, for two or three hours daily, and in the loudest possible tone, will be productive of the greatest advantage in strengthening their voice, and bringing it under their command. There is this benefit in this practice, that it does not keep the attention fixed upon the impediment. In the discipline of the organs, if they can obtain any one to assist them it will be all the better. They should habituate their organs to the pronunciation of those sounds which they find most difficult. The consonants alone, and in combination, will require most attention, and the pupil's friend must remind him when he is wrong. He should pronounce the difficult sounds for him, and let him see the way in which these are pronounced. The false motions of the tongue, lips, etc., must be corrected, and they must learn the proper position of these organs. Great care must be taken to keep the mouth well open, and to make no attempt to speak when the lips are too near together. The lips should never be forcibly compressed, they should but slightly touch, and immediately be brought apart as if with a rebound. Singers are instructed to keep their mouths constantly open, wide enough to admit two fingers between the teeth. Now, it is not meant of course, that they should not close their lips, because then it would be impossible to articulate; but only that they should commence with their mouths fairly open, touch the lips and teeth together only when required for the formation of labials and dentals, and instantaneously bring them back to the former position. This rule must be observed by the stammerer. He must separate his lips or teeth at the very instant they touch; and their resting place must be at some distance apart.

The pupil when he wishes to speak, must first place himself in a position perfectly easy and natural. The next thing is to open his mouth—for he cannot speak without his mouth is open. His third object is to obtain command of sound. The utterance of a vowel, or commencing a hum, will serve to open the glottis, and give him a command of voice. This should be done in a manner perfectly easy and natural, and without the least effort. If an effort is made, the patient draws in his breath, and the attempt at utterance takes place in this situation—with the breath stopped. Having the command of sound, he can speak freely. Hence the importance of attending to the method of inhalation. The gradual and gentle emission of sound should be practised. We have already seen that much benefit may be derived from learning to sing. Besides, the peculiar mode of articulation in singing, singers learn to prolong a note to an almost indefinite extent. This practice will form an excellent exercise for the stammerer. Every public speaker might derive many valuable hints from the art of singing, and it is now allowed that any person may learn to sing, with sufficient time and pains. A musical ear is not so necessarily the gift of nature, as was formerly believed. If not possessed, it may be acquired. Therefore I recommend every stammerer to learn to sing. To return to inhalation: the patient must be very careful to avoid sudden and forcible attempts at inspiration and expiration. The air should be taken in without effort, and allowed to pass out in a slow and continued current. The practice of taking long breaths is beneficial, but these long breaths must be taken without effort, and without allowing any sound of respiration to be heard. The moment the lungs are expanded to such a degree as to produce inconvenience, inspiration must be stopped, and the moment expiration becomes painful, it should be carried no further. But by practice, the power of husbanding the breath, and prolonging the emission of sound, may be carried to a great extent. By the practice of filling the lungs, and carrying the expansion of the chest as far as it will go without effort and inconvenience, the expansibility and fulness of the chest may, in time, be much increased. It should always be done slowly, and without allowing the breath to be heard. The bad effect of inhaling with effort or carrying inhalation too far, is that a spasmodic action is induced, the air is expired in irregular and convulsive jets. By slow inhalation, the muscles do not become fatigued, but preserve their power to modify the emission of air. They are kept under the control of the will, and can be made to prevent the chest contracting too rapidly. A sentence should always be pronounced without inter-ruption from taking breath. When the pupil first practices this, he can make short sentences, allowing himself places of rest where the sense will permit. But in a short time he will acquire the art of prolonging sound indefinitely: pronouncing the longest sentences without perceptible interruption from breathing. The air is taken into the lungs spontaneously, and the current of sound passes steadily on. The lungs are filled sufficiently between the imperceptible pauses in the emission of sound, for the purpose both of voice and of vital action.

In addition to these objects of attention; to wit, to place himself in an easy position, to keep his mouth well open, to obtain command of voice, the only remaining one is the management of the lips and tongue. On this I have already spoken sufficiently. He must acquire this power by imitation where it is possible, and where it is not—where he cannot obtain assistance, he will find directions in books on elocution, for the articulation of the elementary sounds. His practice should be conducted before a glass.

The rapid results produced by the system called Mrs. Leigh's, I have said were real. They were made, and can be made as speedily as I have declared. But though the cures appear perfect for the time, until they are confirmed by long habit, there is great danger of a relapse. In a few cases, they will remain permanent, but in a majority, unless the course is persisted in, the difficulty returns. Moreover, if the affection is produced as I have said by mental causes, as long as those causes remain in the mind unchecked, they will be constantly acting to reproduce the disease. *Causa non sublata, non tollitur effectus.*

Liability to embarrassment, or to be carried away by strong emotion, will constantly operate to produce a recurrence of stammering. Now this disease is, different from all others, for the moment the patient who has imagined himself cured, hears himself stammer, he loses confidence; the fear of stammering returns, and causes him to stammer in his next attempt at utterance. Perfect self command, is, therefore, all important.

Whatever method may be employed for the relief of this affection, no permanent advantage will be gained, in the majority of cases, unless resolutely persevered in for one or two years. With this perseverance, it may be cured with as much certainty as any other chronic disorder, and this not by any new or patent method, but simply by attention to the course I have described.

Boston, August, 1837

SURVEY OF PATENTED
ANTI-STUTTERING DEVICES

MURRAY KATZ

Council of Adult Stutterers, 11435 Monterrey Drive, Silver Spring, Maryland 20902

Various types of devices have been patented to alleviate stuttering. Some prevent certain physical actions, such as clamping of the teeth, improper movement of the tongue and improper breathing. Others strengthen or incapacitate certain muscles. The devices and their alleged action on the body are described. United States as well as foreign patents are included. No attempt has been made to evaluate said devices.

Most stutterers, during and preceding a block, interfere with the normal action of their articulating members so as to render themselves incapable of speaking fluently. They may clench their teeth, press the tongue against the teeth or roof of the mouth, try to speak while inhaling and/or have muscles go into spasm. These actions may be avoidance patterns, which are not part of the true elementary block, but which the stutterer has developed in his attempts to cover up the moment of blockage. Many times these avoidance patterns are so deeply engrained and so automatic that the stutterer is not even aware of them.

Inventors have taken these concepts into consideration and developed devices, which according to described operation, will counteract or modify the action of certain articulating members, exercise and strengthen certain muscles or at least make the stutterer more aware of what he is doing with his articulating members so as to allow speech to be possible. Some of the devices are meant to be used at all times, while others are exercise devices and are used during training periods only. Thus, the device of Bates, which is a tube-like member, remains in the mouth at all times to allow passage of air, while the device of Beattie is clearly for training purposes only, its size and effect on the mouth being ludicrous in addition to preventing normal speech.

A number of these devices have a psychological rather than a physical effect on the stutterer. Thus, the Klein apparatus depends on the well known principle that most stutterers can usually speak fluently when they are alone or when distracting noises are present. Klein provides background noise so that the stutterer cannot hear himself when he is speaking.

This survey of patents includes U.S. as well as foreign patents.

No evaluation of any of the devices has been made since their effectiveness has not been tested. In fact, it is not even known whether any of these devices have been manufactured and been made available. It will be noted that many of the descriptions set forth theoretical concepts which may encourage further experimentation. Is it true, for example, as stated by Conway, that the hyo-glossus muscle is very weak in stutterers? If affirmative, does strengthening of this muscle lead to greater fluency?

These devices have been categorized according to type of function. It is interesting to see how different inventors have approached the problem.

A. DEVICES WHICH KEEP THE AIR PASSAGES OPEN EVEN WHEN THE TEETH ARE CLENCHED AND THE TONGUE IS PRESSED AGAINST THE ROOF OF THE MOUTH.

1. Bates, U.S. 8,394, September 30, 1851.

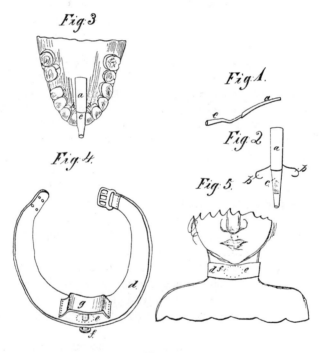

Fig. A-1.

A tube extends the length of the tongue and passes between the lips. The action is described as allowing free passage of air even when the tongue is pressed against the roof of the mouth or teeth and speech is prevented by an undue or spasmodic action of the muscles tending to stop the air. The extension of the tube between the lips prevents closure even when the lips are compressed.

2. Blum, German No. 450,872, October 12, 1927.

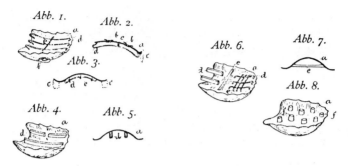

Fig. A-2.

The devices fit against the roof of the mouth. They contain grids or projections to space the tongue therefrom and allow free passage of air, even when the tongue is pressed to the roof of the mouth.

3. Knoch, Br. No. 16,045, July 16, 1906.

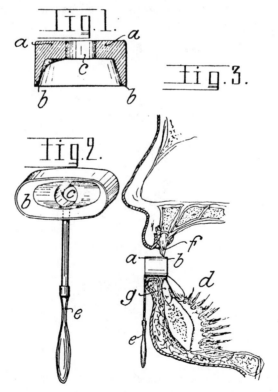

Fig. A-3, B-1.

A device is inserted between the teeth. It is perforated so as to allow free utterance of speech even when the teeth are clenched. The instrument is oval and dished to accommodate the tongue. It has a handle to enable the patient to hold the instrument during conversation.

B. DEVICES WHICH PREVENT THE CLENCHING OF THE TEETH BY THE USE OF A FLEXIBLE SPACER OR SPRING ACTIVATED MEANS TO MAINTAIN THE UPPER AND LOWER TEETH APART, OR TO REQUIRE EXTRA EFFORT TO MOVE THE JAWS TOGETHER. THESE, BY FAR, COMPRISE THE MOST COMMON PATENTED ARTICLES.

1. Knoch, Br. No. 16,045, July 16, 1906.

This patent, described before in connection with devices which allow air passage, also describes the apparatus as preventing

> convulsive closing of the upper and lower rows of teeth . . . which is the chief—if not the sole—condition necessary for the cure of stuttering. By degrees the stutterer learns instinctively and so to say automatically to keep the two rows of teeth apart and the use of the instrument is then no longer necessary.

2. Monday, U.S. 584,696, June 15, 1897.

Fig. 1.

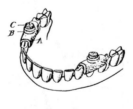

Fig. 2.

Fig. B-2.

U-Shaped clips are placed on one or more teeth. The clips have sockets for holding a pad of soft material, such as rubber, which comes in contact with the opposite jaw. The function is described as follows:

Its presence between the jaws creates, as will be readily understood, a tension of the masseter muscles, whereby the spasmotic action from which arises the imperfection or impediment of speech is overcome or prevented. It is designed to create a permanent cure in a short time.

3. Warnecke, Germany 186,348, June 18, 1907.

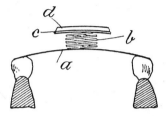

Fig. B-3.

This device, in addition to inhibiting complete closure of the mouth, is designed to prevent the tongue from moving forward to touch the gums when the mouth is substantially closed. The device comprises a bridge-like member which rests on the lower side teeth. Attached to the top middle portion thereof is a spring, the spring having a rubber suction cup at the upper end. The rubber adheres to the roof of the mouth.

4. Hausstein, Ger. 255,645, January 14, 1913. (See Fig. B-4).

This device has a portion to be gripped by the teeth. A flange having ball members at the lower end extends under the tongue and holds it up and in movable position.

The theory is that cramping or fixation of the tongue and face muscles is avoided. The stutterer is said to have a light touch on consonants and achieves self control and confidence.

5. Beattie, U.S. 1,030,965, July 2, 1912. (See Fig. B-5)

This device fits into the mouth and holds the articulating organs so they cannot act at all. As described by the inventor:

the instrument is so arranged that it will bind the articulating organs, namely, jaws, tongue, and lips, at a widely separated position and so that they cannot act at all, even to a slight degree. The purpose of rendering these organs inactive is primarily to prohibit the nervous energy in the brain from entering the motor nerve centers of the articulating organs at all, and, on the other hand, to turn such energy entirely into the motor centers of the vocal organism, namely, the larynx and diaphragm. The sending of such large and abnormal amounts of energy through these last named motor centers and neural processes (under the guidance of one who understands neurology and the neural nature of stammering, stuttering, and normal speech) opens up the vocal processes in the brain to such a degree of previousness that they will complete successfully for the bulk of the speech energy and carry it safely away from the articulating processes and organs, which is the primary object of our invention.

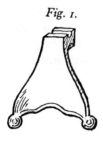

Fig. 1.

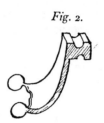

Fig. 2.

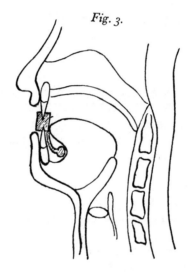

Fig. 3.

Fig. B-4.

Adjustable features allow giving freedom to less troublesome organs, while keeping the more troublesome organs inactive.

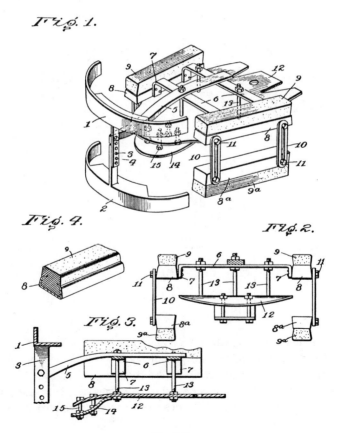

Fig. B-5.

6. Peate, U.S. 1,030,964, July 2, 1912.

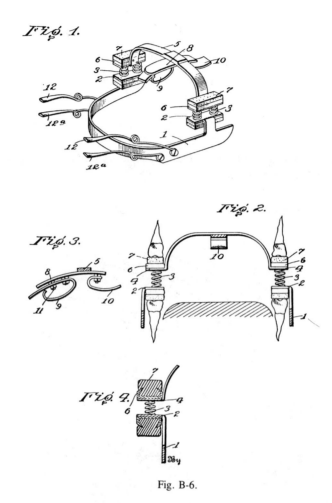

Fig. B-6.

The device is to be used when the patient has gained sufficient control after using the Beattie 1,030,965 device. This device also fits in the mouth but is less cumbersome. It does not immovably fix the lips, tongue and jaws. The action is described as exerting certain pressures on these organs of speech and controlling the patient's speech energy as it divides itself and is distributed to the various organs.

The next series of patents may be grouped together since they describe devices which have biting plates and spring means to keep the plates apart. The springs function to require the patient to exert a stronger effort at pronunciation. The more precise speaking reduces stuttering.

7. Warnecke, Ger. 186,347, June 18, 1907.

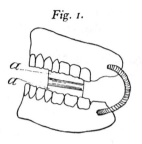

Fig. 1.

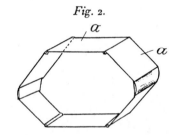

Fig. 2.

Fig. B-7.

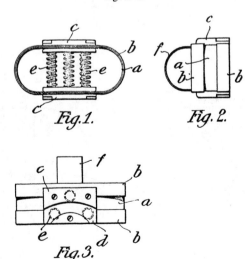

Fig. 1.   Fig. 2.

Fig. 3.

Fig. B-8.

Closure of the mouth is inhibited by a rubber covered hexagonal tubular spring-like device which fits in the mouth. The device allows the tongue to fit in the hollow area and exerts pressure on the roof and floor of the mouth. Complete cure of stuttering is claimed.

8. Warnecke, Ger. 206,652, February 8, 1909.

The spring is directly between the plates, and a handle is provided for holding the device.

9. Kackell, Ger. 330,469, December 16, 1920.

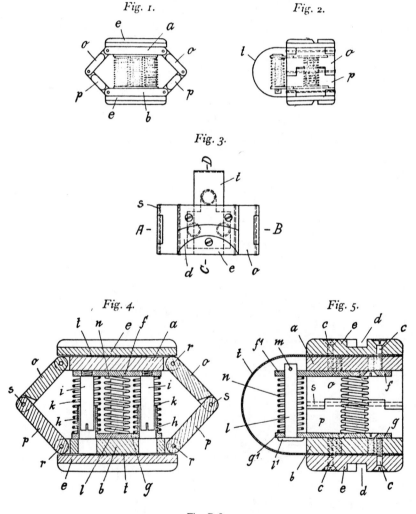

Fig. B-9.

This device is similar to that of Warnecke, Ger. 206,652 and provides an improvement in that the biting plates are kept from twisting when pressed together by the teeth.

10. Voss, Ger. 518,674, February 7, 1930.

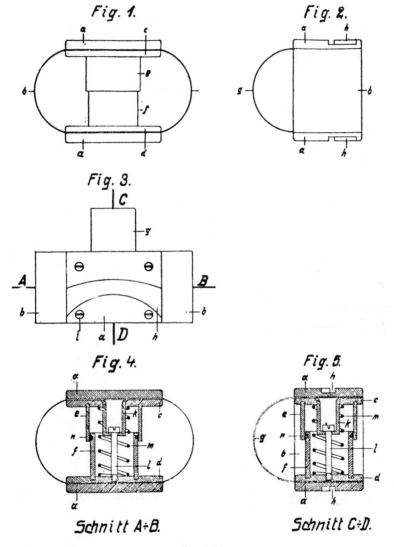

Fig. B-10.

Sleeves protect the springs and serve as guides to prevent twisting.

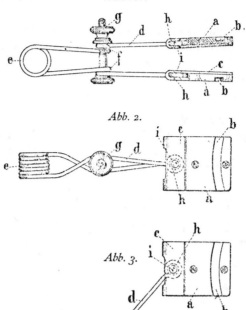

Abb. 1.

Abb. 2.

Abb. 3.

Fig. B-11.

Abb. 1.

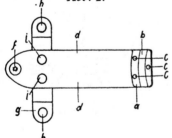

Abb. 3.

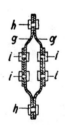

Abb. 2.

Abb. 4.

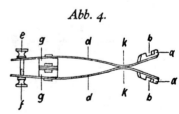

Fig. B-12.

11. Hautau, Ger. 392,002, March 19, 1924.

An externally mounted spring is used, which spring swings out of the way to allow the wearer to read.

12. Pischetsrieder, Ger. 432,002, July 28, 1926.

The tension of the externally mounted spring may be adjusted and provides a portion against which the lips may rest.

13. Steinmeier, Ger. 521, 599, March 25, 1931.

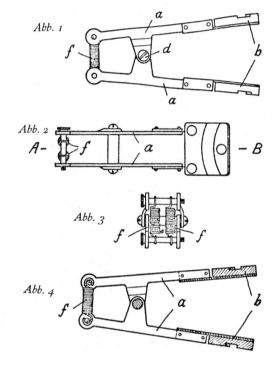

Fig. B-13.

A spring-biased hinged frame in which the springs may be changed to modify the pressure.

14. Stelz, U.S. 2,549,398, April 17, 1951.

Pressure is maintained against the teeth by mouthpieces to make the patient exert a slightly stronger effort at pronunciation than is normally required. This is said to cause the patient to bring the whole orifice of the mouth into full and coordinated action and thereby correct stuttering.

A number of adjustable springs bias the mouthpieces apart. As correction of stuttering takes place the spring action is weakened.

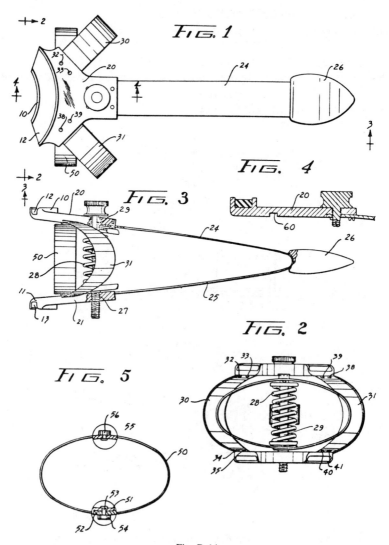

Fig. B-14.

C. DEVICES WHICH EXERCISE OR SUPPRESS THE ACTION OF CERTAIN MUSCLES.

1. Rogers, U.S. 1,327,407, January 6, 1920.

A curved plate, having its greatest thickness in the center, is placed between the lower lip and teeth and is described as

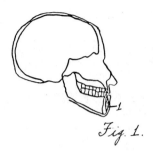

Fig. 1.

Fig. 2.

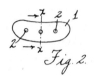

Fig. 3. Fig. 4.

Fig. C-1.

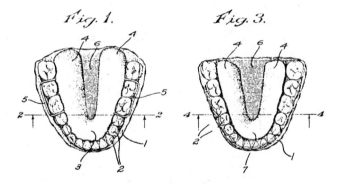

Fig. 1. Fig. 3.

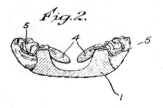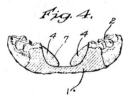

Fig. 2. Fig. 4.

Fig. C-2.

having the function of changing the conformation of the lower lip and placing the muscles known as *depressor labii inferioris*, under tension thus eliminating the involuntary action of the muscles in the spasm of stammering.

This device is characterized as being entirely hidden from view when in use and as not interfering with articulation.

2. Conway, U.S. 1,556,493, October 6, 1925.

The device is stated as exercising the *hyo-glossus muscle* of the tongue, which is, according to the inventor, very weak in stutterers. The hyo-glossus muscle forms the under surface and part of the body of the tongue.

The device for strengthening this muscle comprises a bifurcated member, somewhat V-shaped, adapted to fit within the lower jaw and positioned inside the row of teeth and to lie substantially horizontal under the tongue with the furcations extending rearwardly. The furcations present a smooth inclined surface to the under portion of the tongue. The center portion of the tongue is not inhibited from free movement.

3. Roben, U.S. 1,806,919, May 26, 1931.

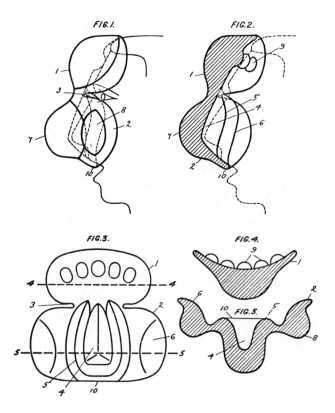

Fig. C-3.

The inventor believes that stutterers and other poor speakers strain the neck muscles leaving the face muscles inactive or not properly controlled. By the use of a face mask, having a number of projections, certain muscles are irritated and caused to contract causing them to operate the resonating cavities. The user gradually acquires the ability to control the involved muscles without the mask.

The mask catches and lifts the upper lip of the wearer and the projections press the muscles on the side of the nose, the cheek muscles and the muscles of the forehead. The muscles of the neck are released from tension.

4. Glisson, U.S. 2,098,867, November 9, 1937.

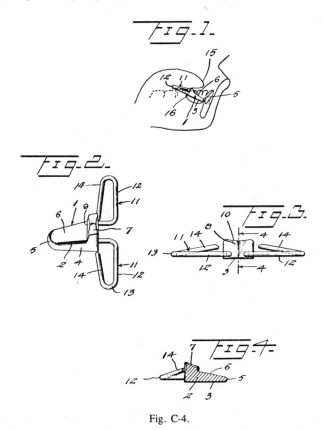

Fig. C-4.

This device is placed in the mouth under the tongue. It rests against and pushes back against the frenum, while the tip of the tongue has free movement. In the words of the patent,

"The—device—will suppress the action of the muscles of the mouth which are responsible for stammering or stuttering speech."

5. Messine, U.S. 2,505,056, April 25, 1950.

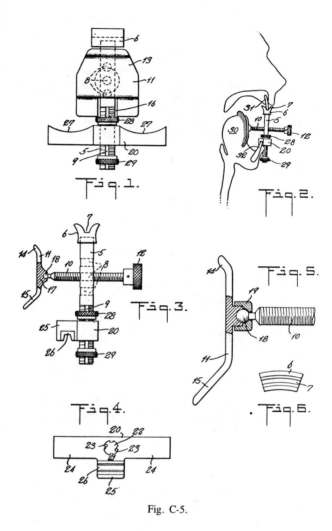

Fig. C-5.

This device consists of a mouth prop, by which the mouth may be held open, in combination with a rod, which serves to hold a tongue support to push the tongue back horizontally in a straight line. In this way the muscles of the tongue, jaw and larynx, essential to phonation are activated, while the muscles normally employed for mastication are freed.

Among many speech defects, stuttering is said to be eradicated.

6. Samual, British 10,256, A.D. 1913.

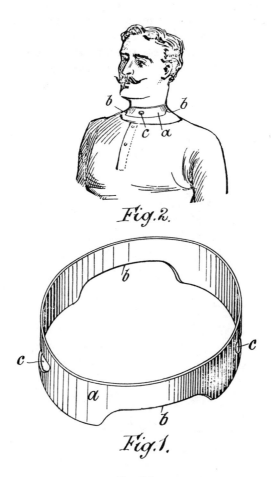

Fig. C-6.

An elastic neck band functions to cause the muscles of the throat and the nerves so stimulated to be strengthened during breathing, speaking and swallowing. The habit of stammering is said to be remedially affected.

D. DEVICES WHICH ALLOW BETTER CORRELATION BETWEEN BREATHING AND SPEAKING.

1. Izuhura, British 501,779, March 6, 1939.

A device is attached to the upper palate in the mouth. It has a double function. A reed produces a "pilot sound" when activated by the air of expiration. This allows the person to be fully conscious of the respiratory movements, and to allow him to begin speaking when breathing out. The sound of the reed is said to give the stutterer confidence. The device also has a sharp projection for pricking the tongue when it is pressed against the palate and is intended to prevent incorrect movements of the tongue.

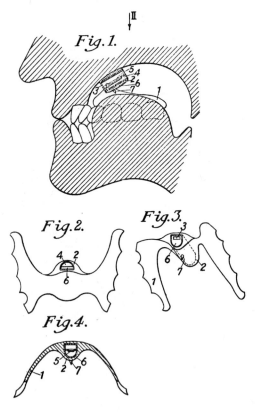

Fig. D-1.

2. Uchiumi, Germany 645,071, May 21, 1937.

This device is worn around the chest. As the chest expands during inhalation a first member forces a plunger against a spring. Further expansion causes the first member to slip out of position. This allows the plunger, under the action of the spring, to prod the chest of the stutterer and remind him that he has adequate breath to begin speaking.

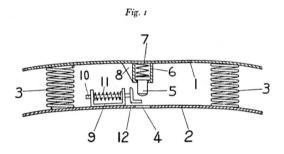

Fig. 1

Fig. 2

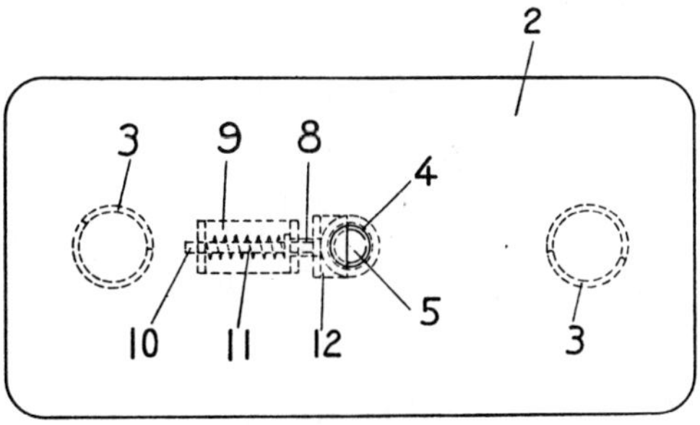

Fig. D-2.

3. Azaretti, Swiss 218,761, April 16, 1942.

A pressure gauge, consisting of a balloon and a meter, are strapped to encircle the torso. By reading the meter, the stutterer can observe his breathing and can improve his breathing and learn to speak at the proper time.

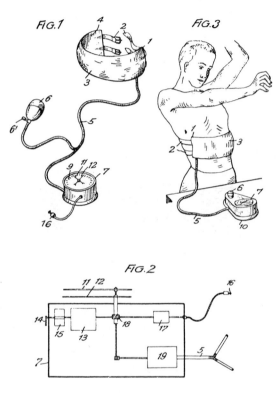

Fig. D-3.

E. MISCELLANEOUS DEVICES.

These patents are put into a common group not because they are less important, but only because there are very few in each category.

1. Use of a weight on tongue to insure slow speech. Gardner, U.S. 625,879, May 30, 1899.

A slotted V-shaped metal piece is clamped over the tongue. The weight of the clamp forces the wearer to speak slowly and to enunciate distinctly.

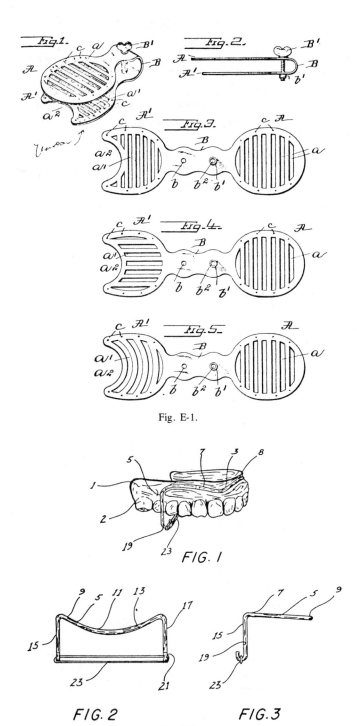

Fig. E-1.

FIG. 1

FIG. 2

FIG. 3

Fig. E-2.

2. A method of interrupting the tongue to break the reflex habit of the stutterer. Freed, U.S. 2,818,065, December 31, 1957.

A wire device fits over the top gums and has downwardly extending legs which extend down toward the teeth. An elastic member is fastened to the legs and extends across the oral cavity to present mechanical interference with the movements of the tongue.

The device slows the speech movement and requires conscious effort for clear enunciation. The reflex habit of stuttering is said to be broken.

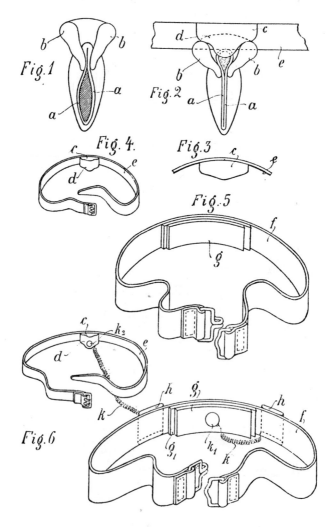

Fig. E-3.

3. Devices to open the glottis. Melzer, British 9, 825, A.D. 1908. Melzer, Sweden 28,596, May 30, 1908.

Since the British patent is more detailed, discussion will be limited thereto.

The apparatus functions to close the glottis since "stammering only takes place when the glottis is open."

The glottis is closed by means of a neck band, which has a pad to push apart the arytenoid cartilages, which in turn causes the glottis to close.

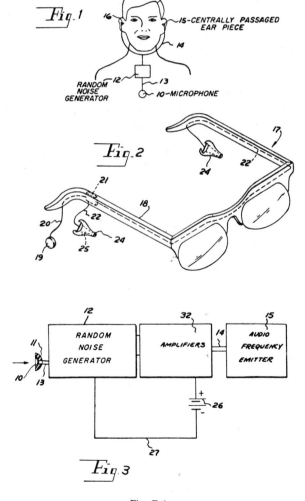

Fig. E-4.

A body belt member is used to apply a pad containing a soothing chemical (oil of cloves) to the body to sooth the nerves.

Electric current may be run between the neck pad, the body pad and the body to "increase the action" of the pads.

Incidentally, it is noted that Bates, U.S. 8,394 states the opposite. Bates employs a neck strap to press the glottis or larynx to an open position. However, since the devices are similar, it is probable that the effect on the glottis is the same.

4. Use of masking noise. Klein, U.S. 3,349,179, October 24, 1967.

The stutterer wears an earpiece which is attached to a random noise generator. The generator is activated by a microphone switch only when the stutterer speaks. The theory is that the stutterer will find relief when he cannot hear his own voice. The earpiece is apertured to allow sound from sources other than the stutterer's own voice to enter his ears.

Summary

The description of these antistuttering devices has been available for many years. It would be interesting to know how many have actually been manufactured, how many have been put into use, and how valid the theories are when put into practice.

INDEX